DISCARD

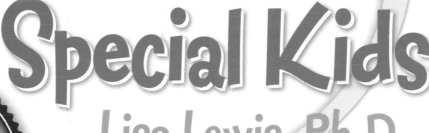

Special Diets
for
Special Kids

Volumes 1 & 2 combined

Lisa Lewis, Ph.D.

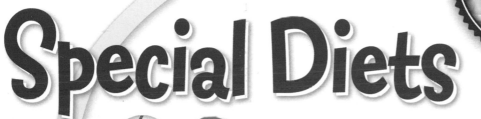

W9-ALZ-827

FUTURE HORIZONS INC.
ARLINGTON, TEXAS

All marketing and publishing rights guaranteed to and reserved by:

FUTURE HORIZONS • 721 W. Abram Street • Arlington, TX 76013
Toll-free: 800-489-0727 • Phone: 817-277-0727 • Fax: 817-277-2270
Website: www.FHautism.com • E-mail: info@FHautism.com

Cover and interior design © TLC Graphics, www.TLCGraphics.com
Cover: Tamara Dever; Interior: Monica Thomas

Photos courtesy of Lisa Lewis, iStockPhoto.com and BigStockPhoto.com

Publisher's Cataloging-In-Publication-Data
(Prepared by The Donohue Group, Inc.)

Lewis, Lisa S.
Special diets for special kids / Lisa Lewis. -- [Rev. and exp. ed.]
p. : col. ill. ; cm. + 1 CD.

"Volumes 1 & 2 combined."
Includes bibliographical references and index.
ISBN: 978-1-935274-12-4

1. Diet therapy for children. 2. Autism--Diet therapy. 3. Gluten-free diet--Recipes.
4. Casein-free diet--Recipes. I. Title.

RJ506.A9 L495 2011
615.854

This book is dedicated to my father,
Leonard Lewis.
I miss him every day.

Table of Contents

Table of Contents *(continued)*

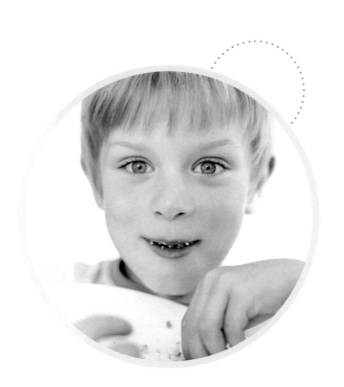

Acknowledgments

A book like this always requires input from many people. At Future Horizons, Kelly Gilpin has been the impetus for this new edition and has calmly encouraged and supported me, even as we listened to the whooshing sound of deadlines passing. Kim Fields has an incredible eye for detail, and caught many errors and omissions in the text and recipes. It is really tedious to read recipes when you are not actually cooking, and I truly appreciate her efforts.

Much of the research for this book was done last year, while I was writing *The Encyclopedia of Dietary Intervention for Autism and Related Disorders* with Karyn Seroussi. Karyn's intellect, work ethic, and support made both these books possible. She has been a valued friend and collaborator for over a decade. Members of the Autism Research Institute conference community have also provided information and articles that helped me complete this edition of *Special Diets*.

Charlie Fall is another supportive friend who has helped me in innumerable ways.

Through her work with the parents of children using dietary intervention, Charlie has learned a lot about what parents need and has passed that on to me. I believe her input (as well as some of her recipes) has made this a better book.

Others who work with parents have been kind enough to share recipes. While they are all acknowledged in the head notes of their recipes, I would like to especially thank Nadine Gilder, Pamela Ferro, and Julie Matthews.

As always, my family has been patient when I was busy writing, and has tasted new recipes without complaint. Serge, Sam, and Jake know that I love them, but I may not always show how much I appreciate them. Thank you all so much.

While many people have read and commented on this book, any mistakes or misstatements are mine.

Lisa Lewis,
March 2011

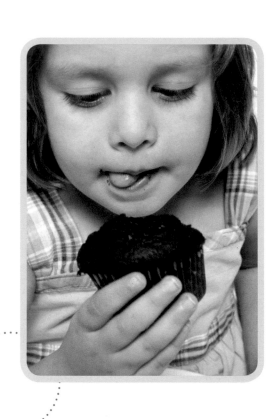

Foreword

BY DR. ELIZABETH MUMPER

Did you know that listening to how your cake crackles and pops during the baking process gives you clues about its level of moisture? Despite being raised in the South, I had never heard of this trick until I read this book — just the latest of many valuable lessons I have learned from Lisa Lewis over the years.

A pediatrician with over twenty-five years of clinical and teaching experience, I started my own practice when I became concerned by the increasing prevalence of autism and other neurodevelopmental disorders. Lisa Lewis's insights have been enormously helpful in this endeavor. As a clinician, I depend on *Special Diets for Special Kids* volumes 1 and 2 for information and recipes for families who come to my center seeking help for their children. As a former medical director of the Autism Research Center, I have welcomed Lisa's valuable contributions to many conferences, workshops, and think tanks. Her wealth of knowledge about diet and autism comes from her own experiences as the mother of a child with autism as well as the collective experience of many other parents who have turned to the Autism Network for Dietary Intervention (ANDI) that she developed with her friend Karyn Seroussi.

Those who have not seen children with autism have major meltdowns after dietary infractions of gluten or casein may be skeptical that diet can play such a major role in behavior. However, many parents have witnessed dramatic improvements in their children's behavior by removing foods that cause harm from their children's diets. They often report to clinicians like me that they see their children regress significantly when these special diets are broken. I believe that it is crucial to spread the word that many (if not most) children with autism can improve with careful attention to nutrition.

Many people still think of food mainly as calories. They have learned that food is separated into categories like proteins, carbo-hydrates, and fats, or food groups like fruits, vegetables, and grains. I invite you to consider food as sources of *information* for the body. For example, nuts and seeds containing magnesium convey calming messages that can benefit symptoms like anxiety, tics, or twitches. Sources of vitamin D instruct your immune system to fight infection, your bones to develop sturdy matrixes, and your cells to regulate signaling patterns. Brightly colored fruits and vegetables bring anti-oxidants to capture free radicals and decrease the chronic oxidative stress many children with autism experience.

This book provides delicious ways to package the benefits food can provide for children with neurodevelopmental disorders. Lisa has compiled a set of recipes that are not only kid friendly, but also easy to prepare. Her carefully gathered dishes, which come from a wide range of cultures, are suitable for all sorts of occasions. Lisa has a talent for explaining the scientific basis of digestive and absorptive problems in autistic children in ways that are easy for overwhelmed parents to understand, and her short anecdotes at the beginning of many of the recipes make for entertaining reading.

When I teach other doctors how to evaluate and treat medical problems found in children with autism, I admonish them to listen to the parents. Now, I encourage you to listen to the wisdom of a mother and writer who has been through the challenges and rewards of cooking in special ways for special children. Whether you are the parent or relative of a recently diagnosed child looking for explanations on how to get started, or the caregiver for a child who has already benefited from dietary interventions and are looking for new recipes, you will find help in this book. Listen to Lisa: she will teach you how to cook creatively in new ways to help the special child in your life.

Introduction

When I began writing the first edition of *Special Diets for Special Kids* in 1998, the world of gluten- and casein-free cooking was a lonely, sparsely populated place. There were few packaged foods available; getting the ingredients for recipes I adapted required a trip to the health food store. Now the gluten-free landscape has been completely transformed. There are so many gluten-free (GF) foods available at the grocery store in my (very small) New Jersey town, I can buy almost everything I need without special trips or Internet vendors. Even my store's "soup bar" has a daily selection that is designated gluten-free! This development is wonderful for anyone who follows (or cooks for someone on) a GF diet.

Likewise, when my book was first published, it was virtually the only one of its type. There were few books for GF diets; for example, the late Bette Hagman's "Gluten-Free Gourmet" books were lifesavers for celiacs and others who needed to avoid gluten. But even these wonderful cookbooks failed to exclude dairy or soy. Today there are dozens of cookbooks available for those on **gluten-free/casein-free (GFCF)** diets — enter these terms on Amazon.com, and you may be overwhelmed with choices.

Given this new environment, one might ask if a new version of *Special Diets for Special Kids* is even necessary. I mean, why not rest on my cookbook laurels and let others do the heavy lifting? This is a question I pondered long and hard before deciding that I did want to spend the time and effort to update the two *Special Diets* books. For one thing, I know a lot more about dietary intervention for autism than I did 12 years ago, and my perspective has changed a lot. Because I have been around, writing and speaking on this topic for years, many people have heard my name and might be drawn to my book. When that happens, I want them to be buying a book with updated information and recipes that reflect recent knowledge and research. I also want to combine the best of both volumes of *Special Diets* into one easy-to-use book. No more "Which volume was that recipe in?" or "Which book should I buy?" quandaries!

It is now clear that it is important to feed our families more naturally, using organic and locally grown foods whenever possible. Because I want to encourage parents to use fewer starches and more nutrient-dense fruits, vegetables, and proteins, I have removed many recipes and have added many new ones. Hopefully, most of these recipes will appeal to even the pickiest eaters. I also want to address an issue that is often raised: "I cannot afford to put my child on a GFCF diet." Anyone can afford to do this, especially when you consider the cost of ignoring your child's diet. Over the years, I have learned lots of tricks for doing the diet "on the cheap," and I want to share them with others.

When my family started following a GFCF diet, I was already an experienced home cook and baker. I assumed that the "hard" part of this diet was baking, and that most readers would already know the basics of cooking. For that reason, I concentrated on recipes that would duplicate the typical American child's diet, and replace all the "goodies" that children on a special diet might miss. However, I now realize that many parents do not have the time to really learn to cook, and when a GFCF diet is suggested, they panic! They are sure that they will be tied to the stove, cooking and baking for hours each day.

The fact is that the easiest (and cheapest) way to go GFCF is to forgo many of the baked goods and stick to simple foods, prepared simply. While the baked foods are great for treats, our children would be better off if they learned to eat fewer carbohydrates. Grilled or broiled chicken beats breaded and fried nuggets from you-know-where any day! For those parents who missed some of the basics — like how to roast a turkey or make a stew — this version of *Special Diets* will tell you how. And because both time and energy can be in short supply, I will include many time- and effort-saving ideas such as making a Thanksgiving turkey in an hour and getting your children to drink their vegetables (and love them).

As I did in the earlier editions of the *Special Diets* books, I have annotated many recipes with "head notes." I did this to share ideas, variations, and tips. Sometimes there is a story that goes with a particular recipe, or a suggestion for how to serve it. I have also included ways to adapt particular recipes for those who are avoiding all starches (e.g., those on the Specific Carbohydrate Diet [SCD]) or who are avoiding particular ingredients. I also point out the benefits of many specific ingredients.

If you are new to dietary intervention, I hope that this book will ease you into the GFCF diet with minimal stress. If you are an old hand, I hope you will find that there are still things you can learn to make life as delicious and nutritious as possible!

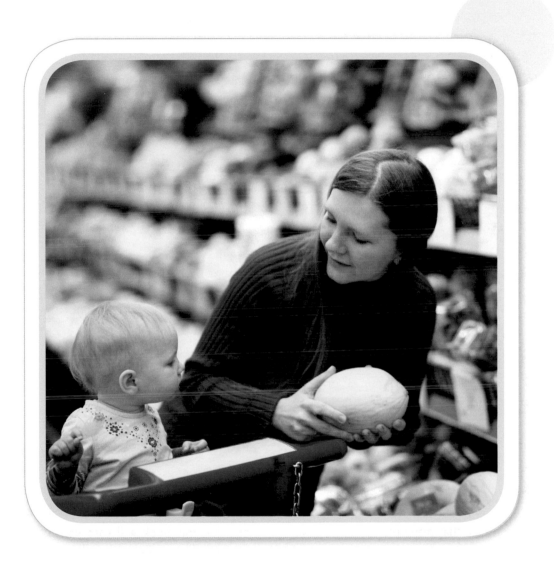

Why Special Diets?

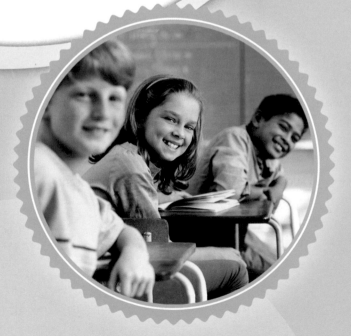

People have used dietary interventions to treat diseases for many years but, as one might expect, this approach is rarely attempted when more conventional medical interventions are already available. Bluntly stated, dietary interventions are almost always tried for disorders that are, at the time, incurable. When no pharmaceutical or surgical treatments are available, diets may be tried out of desperation, from the perspective that "We might as well give *this* a shot." And while not all dietary interventions have been

successful, many have produced significant improvement for specific symptoms.

The **ketogenic diet** is a good example of a diet used to treat a medical problem that seems to bear no relation to food or nutrition. Doctors at Johns Hopkins in Baltimore, Maryland, began using an extremely high-fat, low-protein carbohydrate diet to manage seizure disorders 70 years ago. The ketogenic diet lost popularity many years ago but resurfaced in the 1990s when Dr. John Freeman and nutritionist Millicent Kelly (1996) wrote a book on the use and management of the diet. It is again being used at medical centers around the country to control intractable epileptic seizures in patients who do not respond to conventional drug therapy and are not good candidates for surgery.

Another disorder for which dietary interventions have been used is **attention deficit hyperactivity disorder (ADHD)**. Although estimates vary, some reports place the number of school-aged children taking stimulant medication for this disorder at over two million. As is true for most learning and developmental disabilities, boys with this disorder outnumber girls by a ratio of approximately 2:1. These children have various problems, including distractibility, impulsiveness, and hyperactivity. The behaviors associated with this disorder include difficulty remaining seated and paying attention, difficulty obeying instructions, shifting from one uncompleted activity to another, difficulty playing quietly, talking excessively, interrupting, losing things, and being unaware of the consequences of their actions.

Most children with ADHD are placed on stimulant medication. Despite potential risks and over the objections of many parents, some teachers insist that these boisterous children not be allowed in their classroom unless they are medicated.

For parents of ADHD children, Dr. Ben Feingold came along as a white knight in 1975 when he published *Why Your Child Is Hyperactive*. The late Dr. Feingold was a pediatric allergist in San Francisco who claimed that childhood hyperactivity was caused by food dyes, artificial flavorings, and certain preservatives commonly used to increase the shelf life of foods. He pointed out that over 80% of the food additives in our nation's food supply were composed of artificial colors and flavors.

Feingold hypothesized a genetically mediated sensitivity to certain artificial ingredients, citing the direct correlation between the increasing use of additives and the rise in learning and behavior problems. He prescribed a diet that eliminated these items, as well as foods containing the natural chemicals known as salicylates (salicylates are found in almonds, apples, apricots, berries, cherries, cucumbers, grapes, oranges, plums, tangerines, and tomatoes). Members of the Feingold Association have been helping parents of children with ADHD since 1976; for more information visit their website at http://www.feingold.org.

L. M. Pessler and colleagues (2010) at the ADHD Research Center in the Netherlands reported on their pilot study on the effect of diet on physical and sleep problems commonly seen in ADHD. A group of twenty-seven children were randomly assigned to a diet group or a control group. The diet group followed a 5-week elimination diet, while the controls stuck to their regular diet. Parents kept extensive diaries and monitored behavior, physical, and sleep complaints. "The number of physical and sleep complaints was significantly decreased in the diet group compared to the control group." There were significant reductions in the frequency of headaches, stomachaches, excessive thirst, or perspiration, and sleep issues. They concluded that "An elimination diet may be an effective instrument to reduce physical complaints in children with ADHD, but more research is needed to determine the effects of food on (functional) somatic symptoms in children with and without ADHD."

Artificial colors are complex organic compounds derived from petroleum. They are generally cheaper, more stable, and brighter than natural colorings; however, these advantages come at a great cost. According to the Center for Science in the Public Interest (CSPI), artificial colors should be avoided. "Yellow 5, Red 40, and six other dyes cause cancer in animals, are contaminated with cancer-causing chemicals, and may cause allergic reactions and hyperactivity." (See the CSPI's full report on artificial food colorings at http://www.cspinet.org.)

Although tens of thousands of children and adults with attention deficit disorder (ADD) and ADHD have been helped by the Feingold and other diets, mainstream medicine still considers diet to be an "alternative" treatment. Diet is not even listed as a treatment on the website of the Children and Adults with Attention Deficit/Hyperactivity Disorder (CHADD), the largest national support and information network for these disorders.

While mainstream medicine considers dietary intervention to be controversial for the ADD and ADHD population, a special diet is the *only* accepted treatment for **celiac disease (CD)**. Celiac disease, also known as celiac sprue or gluten-sensitive enteropathy,

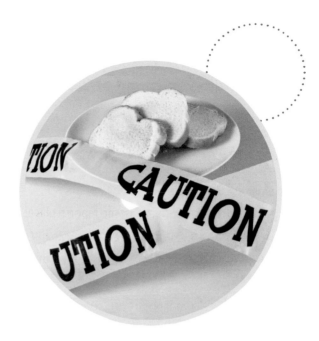

is a chronic disease in which the ingestion of gluten causes a characteristic type of lesion in the small intestine. The destruction of the gut wall causes improper, incomplete nutrient absorption. Children with this disease typically show serious gastrointestinal problems, fatty stools, and slow growth. Research has determined that many patients with a gluten sensitivity serious enough to damage the gut wall *show no digestive symptoms in childhood*; thus, it is likely that there are a great number of undiagnosed celiac children. In CD patients, all sources of gluten must be completely eliminated from the diet.

To fully understand the diet that *must* be used by individuals with celiac disease, and is advocated here for autism and other pervasive developmental disorders, it is important to know what gluten is. Glutens are proteins found in the plant kingdom subclass of *Monocotyledoneae*, the grass family of wheat, oats, barley, rye, and triticale. Derivatives of these grains include malt, grain starches, hydrolyzed vegetable/plant proteins, textured vegetable proteins, grain vinegar, soy sauce, grain alcohol, flavorings, and the binders and fillers found in vitamins and medications.

Why Dietary Intervention for Autism?

Avoiding gluten, and a dairy protein called casein, is at the heart of the dietary interventions outlined in this book. To understand why we need to remove these proteins, it is important to start with some background information about autism research.

The idea of using dietary intervention for autism has its origins in 1980 when neuroscientist Jaak Panksepp observed that children with autism had many traits in common with people addicted to opioid drugs. Addicts are often "in their own world," and frequently exhibit stereotypic behaviors (e.g., rocking). Generally, opiate addicts are insensitive to pain and have serious gastrointestinal problems. Dr. Panksepp (1980) proposed that children with autism might have elevated levels of naturally occurring opioids in their central nervous systems.

These observations led to research in Sweden, Norway, Great Britain, and the United States. In all locations, abnormal peptides were found in the urine of children with autism. These findings ultimately resulted in the postulation of what is now called the "opioid excess theory" of autism. Briefly, this hypothesis suggests that autism and its

associated symptoms may result from the incomplete breakdown of peptides derived from foods that contain gluten and casein, and excessive absorption of these peptides (due to a "leaky gut"). According to the theory's proponents, the presence of these peptides causes disruption to biochemical and neuroregulatory processes in the brain.

At least six independent labs have found abnormal peptides in the urine of children with an autism spectrum disorder (ASD) — peptides that are not found in the urine of typical controls. Clearly something is putting them there. Since removal of foods containing gluten and casein leads to widespread improvement, it makes sense to assume that the foods are the source.

There are strong arguments supporting the removal of gluten and casein. Constipation, self-absorption, and insensitivity to pain are hallmarks of both autism and drug addiction. When these proteins are removed from a child's diet, the physical and emotional withdrawal response can be extreme — simply removing foods to which a person is sensitive should not cause this kind of discomfort. Since it has been shown that the urinary peptides decrease with a GFCF diet, it is reasonable to conclude that they have a dietary origin.

Studies of urine in Norway (Reichelt, 2003), England (Shattock, et al., 1990; Shattock & Whiteley, 2002; Shattock & Whitely, 2006), and the United States (Cade, 2000) all found opioid peptides in the urine of patients with autism. These peptides, primarily from gluten and casein, are close enough

What the Heck Is a Leaky Gut?

In a healthy digestive system, there are small spaces in the lining of the gut. Tiny particles of proteins migrate from the gut into the bloodstream through these spaces. If the gut becomes damaged, its lining may develop larger openings and become too permeable. Such a "leaky" gut may allow polypeptides (chains of amino acids) to pass through the gut into the bloodstream. Incompletely digested foods and toxic fungal waste products can also pass through.

How Does the Intestine Become Too Permeable?

We do not know for sure, but there are several theories. It may be that a viral infection has established itself in the lining of the intestines, disrupting the gut-immune system and weakening the lining. Another theory posits that excessive yeast and/or bacteria has compromised the gut wall. Finally, a genetic predisposition to celiac disease or another allergic reaction in the gut may result in gluten intolerance, flattening the intestinal villi and creating a celiac-like condition. A deficiency in the enzyme phenol sulfur-transferase (PST) may also be to blame because this can cause proteins in the gut lining to stick together and form gaps. Research by Dr. Rosemary Waring (Waring & Ngong, 1993; O'Reilly & Waring, 1993) at the University of Birmingham, UK, has shown that PST deficiency is common in children who have autism. ★

in structure to morphine-class drugs to cause some of the behaviors and symptoms typical of autism spectrum disorders (e.g., self-stimulation, sensory integration disorders, bowel irregularities, insensitivity to pain).

Subsequent research by Alan Friedman and others at Johnson & Johnson (1999) confirmed the presence of these substances in the urine of subjects who have autism. They also found that these subjects were deficient in a digestive enzyme known as Dipeptidyl peptidase-IV (DPP-IV). DPP-IV is the only peptidase that can break apart certain peptides (including opioids).

According to biochemist Jon Pangborn, Ph.D. (2008), some of the children who respond well to dietary intervention may be under the influence of opioids, but they may have other problems as well. For children with weak DPP-IV digestion, opioid peptides that enter the bloodstream could lead to immune system dysregulation. For these children, intestinal inflammation and lesions could result. Digestive enzyme supplements have now been formulated to include this important enzyme.

Related Issues

Research by Dr. Rosemary Waring (1996), of the University of Birmingham, UK, has shown that children diagnosed with an ASD have a marked deficiency in an enzyme group called **phenol sulfur-transferase (PST)**, impairing the body's ability to rid itself of toxins.

During detoxification, toxins are transformed into harmless substances and excreted. The body often accomplishes this transformation by adding a molecule to the toxin, in a process called conjugation. Sulfate conjugation is a process used to transform many chemicals, including environmental toxins, drugs, and neurotransmitters. For this to occur, there must be enough PST. If this enzyme is deficient or there are an insufficient number of sulfate ions, then detoxification is impaired and harmful substances can build up. Some important metabolic processes can also be disturbed by phenolic compounds. PST is also vital to the sulfate conjugation of phenols; this is important because phenolic compounds are nearly everywhere in the environment. Further, if sulfation is deficient, proteins in the gut wall can stick together, causing gaps. In other words, a PST deficiency may contribute to intestinal permeability.

After hearing a talk by Dr. Rosemary Waring on the topic of PST deficiency, Sandra O. Johnson (S. Johnson, 1995) devised **Sara's Diet**. This "white diet" eliminates all artificial and natural pigments to reduce the load on the PST system as completely as possible. Although some foods are eventually returned to the diet, the regimen is extremely restrictive. In Kelly Dorfman's (1997) words: "Some parents have used diets that remove all known phenol compounds (such as Sara's Diet) to take pressure off the PST...system. While sometimes helpful, these diets are extraordinarily difficult to implement long-term as naturally occurring phenols are in every food with color. Except in extreme cases, a diet reducing toxic load from the most concentrated sources...appears to be the best. That is, reduce juices (or limit to pear juice) and eliminate all artificial colors and flavors." As word of PST deficiency spread, many autism researchers were intrigued by the suggestion that it could cause improper metabolism of neurotransmitters. It has been known for years that persons with autism often have abnormal levels of serotonin as measured in the blood. The buildup of serotonin is interesting and may prove to be significant upon further research. Another equally interesting point is the effect a PST deficiency would have on the permeability of the intestinal lining.

Although most of the reports are anecdotal, there is good evidence that a GFCF diet may indeed be extremely beneficial. The opioid peptides in question may stunt normal central nervous system development. Another observation is equally intriguing: "...because most bioactive peptides are found in different chain lengths, but with very similar activity, different peptidase defects would cause similar but not identical symptom profiles and peptide profiles" (Waring & Ngong, 1993). In other words, there could be several different genetic flaws affecting different enzymes that would result in the same symptoms.

What About Yeast?

For the parents of children with developmental delays or disabilities, the medical history often includes a series of ear or respiratory infections and antibiotic treatment. Many parents say their children "practically lived on antibiotics," and many were placed on prophylactic (preventive) doses for periods of months or even years. But while most children fed this diet of antibiotics developed normally, the vast majority of atypical children did ingest the medications, and continued to show, as they matured, severely disordered immune systems.

A basic tenet of allopathic medicine is that infections are due to organisms (bacteria, viruses, or parasites). Organisms can be killed with antibiotics. Therefore, infections should be treated with antibiotics. This view has changed little in the past 50 years despite evidence that the underlying theory is fragmentary and insufficient to explain why we succumb to these organisms. According to Michael Schmidt, Lendon Smith, and Keith Sehnert (1993), doctors simply are not taught alternatives to antibiotic dosing in medical school.

Antibiotic abuse is rampant, even in situations where their usefulness is questionable. Broad-spectrum antibiotics (e.g., Amoxicillin, Keflex, Ceclor, Bactrim, Septra) are most often prescribed for ear infections. Many (if not most) ear infections clear up without treatment. More importantly, these drugs wipe out normal intestinal flora, which can enable the population of normally occurring yeasts to expand dramatically.

When treatment is necessary, doctors sensitive to these problems prescribe drugs such as penicillin or erythromycin, rather than a broad-spectrum drug. Some rare doctors will also prescribe a short course of an antifungal agent such as Nystatin. Obtaining a prescription for an antifungal drug will likely be an uphill battle with most doctors. While they will readily admit that the drugs being prescribed will cause gastrointestinal upsets

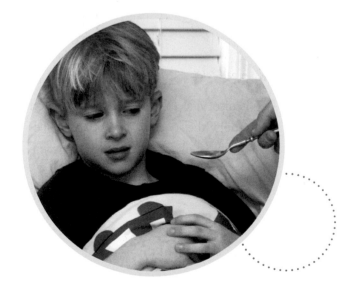

and vaginal yeast infections in women, they still laugh at the notion that an overgrowth of yeast in the gut after taking antibiotics might cause illness.

Many doctors claim that the overuse of antibiotics is the fault of their patients who insist on medicine when they or their children are ill. This is probably true; doctors are not the only ones raised with this model of treatment. However, doctors who knowingly

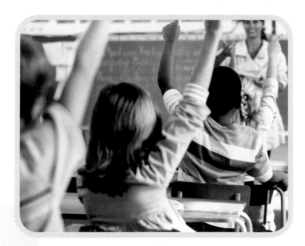

prescribe an antibiotic to treat a viral infection to satisfy a patient's demand are not behaving responsibly. It would only take a few moments to explain that currently available medicines will not help a viral infection, and to suggest some other non-pharmaceutical treatments to alleviate discomfort. If doctors continue to prescribe medications they know will not help a child's illness, it is up to parents to resist the temptation to ask for medication.

In addition to weakening the immune system's ability to recognize and fight off bacterial infection, the abuse of antibiotics has led to strains of antibiotic resistant

bacteria (Schmidt, Smith & Sehnert, 1993). Doctors often must look for new or stronger antibiotics to prescribe for bacterial infections because older ones no longer work.

The late Dr. William Crook of Jackson, Tennessee, long championed the notion that abuse of antibiotics has damaged children. He believed that a vicious cycle begins when an upper respiratory or ear infection is treated with antibiotics. The antibiotic throws off the balance of the intestinal flora by killing off "good" bacteria, which provide protection against fungal and parasitic infections, help break down complex foods, and synthesize certain vitamins. With so many useful (or "friendly") organisms destroyed, yeast (*Candida albicans*) can grow unchecked, causing infections that have many troubling and seemingly unrelated symptoms, and can cause or contribute to the leakiness of the gut. This unhealthy situation leads to more infections, more antibiotics, and...well, you get the idea.

Over the course of his long career, Dr. Crook treated hundreds of children with autism. He repeatedly saw the pattern described above. He pioneered the use of low-sugar diets and antifungal medication, and many children have been helped significantly by his treatment (Crook, 1986). Despite the fact that the majority of mainstream medicine has scoffed at the notion of disease being caused by an organism that naturally occurs in our intestines, improvement is too widespread to dismiss, and other doctors are now looking into the "yeast connection."

Work by Dr. William Shaw, a Kansas City biochemist, has provided additional evidence to support Dr. Crook's long-held theories. Shaw has found unusually high levels of fungal metabolites (yeast waste products) in the urine of several groups of abnormally functioning individuals, including people with autism (Shaw & Kassen, 1995: Shaw, 2008). His first paper describing this phenomenon was published in 1995, and he has conducted many other studies on the effect of antifungal therapy on urinary organic acids on children with autism.

According to Dr. Stephen B. Edelson, as *Candida* proliferates in the gut, it can undergo anatomical and physiological changes to become a different kind of fungus, a mycelial fungus (Edelson, 1997). *Candida*'s original state is non-invasive, but as a mycelial fungus, it produces structures that penetrate mucosal linings and break down the lining between the intestines and the rest of the circulation. In other words, *Candida* infections may also contribute to damage of the gut wall, enabling large molecules to cross the blood-brain barrier. Edelson points out that this damage could be introducing many substances into the blood that should not be there. Thus, it is not surprising that many people with yeast overgrowth also show allergies to foods and environmental substances. Edelson cites work in England and in the United States at the National Institutes of Health (NIH) that supports the notion that "some of these incomplete protein-breakdown products, if absorbed, may have endorphin-like activity and can change mood, mind, memory, and behavior."

Critics of the "yeast connection" syndrome argue that not every illness can be cured by antifungal medication and special diets. This is certainly true. But it is also true that many people, adults as well as children, have been on an antibiotic "merry-go-round" that has damaged their body's ability to heal itself and fight off infections. Anyone who has ever taken erythromycin or doxycycline can attest to the fact that it causes intense gastrointestinal discomfort. Why is it so difficult to accept that these medications do damage, in some people, that outlasts the course of the medication or the illness for which it was prescribed?

Allergies and Intolerances

Many children and adults claim to suffer from food allergies. While most doctors maintain that food allergies are extremely rare, patients often find relief when treated with elimination and rotation diets. Although the incidence of the problem seems to have increased in modern times, its existence was recorded in the time of Hippocrates, who noted that cow's milk could cause hives and stomachaches. "One man's meat is another man's poison" is believed to have been written by the Roman poet Lucretius, and the saying seems to be just as true today.

Of course, no one really doubts that food allergies exist; most people know persons who are unable to eat seafood without a serious reaction. And many children are not allowed to bring peanut products to school because they can provoke a life-threatening anaphylaxis in some children.

The term *allergy* has a specific, medical meaning, but it is often used incorrectly to describe what is really a sensitivity or intolerance. An allergic reaction can be caused by any form of direct contact with an allergen: eating or drinking a food you are sensitive to (ingestion); breathing in pollen, perfume, or pet dander (inhalation); or touching the allergen (direct contact). An *allergen* is any harmless component that causes an adverse reaction involving the immune system.

Classic allergy (also called "Type-I" or "IgE" allergy) refers to the type of allergy in which a reaction is most often immediate. Most Type-I allergic reactions are expressed as hay fever, sneezing, and itching and redness of the eyes. There can be skin reactions such as swelling, itching, or hives. Inhaled allergens can also lead to asthmatic symptoms: shortness of breath, coughing, and wheezing. Sometimes, an allergic reaction to food is confined to the mucus membranes in and around the mouth. Food allergy can also cause stomach pain and/or vomiting. In its most serious presentation, food allergy can be fatal.

According to the American Academy of Family Physicians, about 8% of children and 2% of adults have a Type-I food allergy. Milk allergy is much more common in children than in adults. Children usually outgrow allergies to milk, eggs, soy, and wheat by the time they are 6 years old, but people usually do not outgrow allergies to peanuts, tree nuts, fish, and shellfish.

Many children with autism have classic allergies, but are they more "allergic" than age-matched controls? A recent study found that 30% of the subjects with autism had a family history of classic allergy, compared to only 2.5% of the controls. However, actual prevalence of classic allergy in both groups was not much different. Another study concluded that food allergies and severe constipation are an extremely common finding in children who have autism. Moreover, researchers at the New Jersey Medical School found that there were "intrinsic defects of innate immune responses (to cow's milk protein) in ASD children with gastrointestinal symptoms."

Not as well-understood are IgG allergies (also called "Type-II allergies," "intolerances," or "sensitivities"). These allergies are not life-threatening, and usually present with subtler symptoms, including red cheeks or ears, itchy skin, stomachaches, diarrhea, gas, headaches, joint pain, sleeplessness, or hyperactivity. For some reason, children with autism and their typical siblings tend to have higher values on IgG tests than children in a typical population. Even though most allergists do not place much value on, or test for, IgG reactivity, they will usually acknowledge that foods can cause a reaction or intolerance in some people, even though the reaction is not strictly a classic allergy.

Based on the premise that children with autism have something awry in their immune systems, here are some possibilities as to why children who have autism are more likely to be intolerant to food:

◉ They have a genetic vulnerability to food allergies *and* to the environmental trigger(s) leading to autism.

◉ They have a genetic vulnerability to the environmental trigger(s) leading to autism. The trigger sets off an immune problem that leads to allergy. For example: If the gut-immune system is damaged by a viral insult, the gut lining is weakened, and foods leak into the bloodstream and trigger a sensitivity or an allergic response.

◉ Early exposure to allergens (especially cow's milk) in an allergic infant creates a vulnerability to the environmental trigger(s) leading to autism.

◉ Infants with IgG milk intolerance may be more prone to ear infections, leading to antibiotic use, gut dysbiosis, leaky gut, and food allergy/peptiduria. It is also possible that an IgG gluten intolerance, either inborn or acquired, is responsible for the breakdown of the intestinal lining in some children (analogous to celiac disease). This may explain why some older children, after the gut has healed and the behaviors associated with autism have resolved, will regress several weeks after gluten is re-introduced.

Understanding Gut Dysbiosis

by Elizabeth Mumper, MD, reprinted from *The ANDI (Autism Network for Dietary Intervention) News*.

Working with developmentally disabled children has given me a renewed appreciation for the multiple roles of the gut. In addition to its obvious role in digestion, it functions as a vital barrier that protects our bodies from the harmful effects of what we ingest.

You may know that our intestines form an integral part of our immune systems, but did you also know that the gut, just like the brain, has receptors for many neurotransmitters? These are the chemicals that transmit nerve signals between synapses in the nervous system. Further, our guts support a thriving environment (or flora) of bacteria and yeast. This flora consists of about a quadrillion individual germs, which also live on the skin, eyes, digestive tract, and vagina.

The guts of breast-fed infants are initially colonized with beneficial bacteria, including *lactobacillus* and bifidobacteria. In exchange for a place to live, our gut flora perform many important tasks such as fighting off harmful microbes, manufacturing certain vitamins, and converting food into fuel for the body and brain.

When the delicate balance of the ecosystem in our intestines is disrupted, however, the good bacteria may be depleted. Even a single course of antibiotics can wreak havoc on normal intestinal flora. (Other factors include surgery, gastroenteritis, and other medications.) When harmful flora flourishes, it can produce substances that are biochemically similar to normal neurotransmitters. This is called "molecular mimicry." As these messages are processed, we may suffer from clouded thinking, feel drunk or achy, or develop symptoms that are hard to diagnose. Furthermore, the release of these toxins (often considered microbial "waste products") can interfere with the body's detoxification mechanisms. Our bodies now find it more difficult than ever to handle pollutants, at a time when toxins are being added to our environment at warp speed.

Judicious use of probiotics and intermittent use of *Saccharomyces boulardii*, a good yeast that fights bad yeast, can promote the normal balance of the many bacterial and yeast inhabitants of our guts. Probiotic supplements or cultured foods with active cultures can help re-establish beneficial flora in the intestines.

Children on the autism spectrum seem to be at particular risk for pathogenic bacteria, especially *Clostridium*. Stool analyses can be used to identify and quantify bacteria so that pathogenic species can be identified and treated. For example, *Clostridia* is treated with oral Vancomycin, sometimes in combination with Flagyl or oral gentamicin. Certain children with autism respond positively to treatment with antifungal agents like Diflucan, Sporanox, Lamisil, or Ketoconazole. The reasons for this are still unclear, since studies to date do not demonstrate increased colonies of yeast in children who have autism, compared to controls. Some symptoms to look out for are red rings around the anus, chronic constipation or diarrhea, or a history of multiple courses of antibiotics.

People know that they need to exercise to build muscles, take calcium to maintain their bones, and eat a "heart-healthy" diet to prolong their lifespan. How many of those same people understand how crucial it is to take care of their guts, and the flora that live there symbiotically? Far from being a lowly corridor that simply turns food into waste, our gut performs many vital functions, and needs to be kept healthy in order for us to stay healthy. ★

. . . .

Dr. Elizabeth Mumper is a general pediatrician treating a large number of children with autism and attention problems. She is the former Medical Director of the Autism Research Institute (ARI), CEO of Advocates for Children, and the founder of the RIMLAND Center in Lynchburg, Virginia.

Allergy Testing

Allergies

IgE ("Type I") allergies are most commonly tested for with skin tests and blood tests. In a skin test, a series of needle pricks are made on the patient's skin (usually the patient's back) to introduce small amounts of suspected allergens. If the patient is allergic to a given substance, a visible response (a small welt) will occur, usually within 30 minutes. Positive responses can range from a slight redness to full-blown hives. Any allergist can perform these tests in-office; it usually takes a couple of hours, so bring something to keep your child busy. Do not give your child Benadryl or any other antihistamine for 24 hours before the test; this will invalidate the results.

While skin tests are simple and inexpensive, they are not very accurate. Some people show delayed reactions as long as 6 hours after the tests. The introduction of potential allergens during the test may sensitize some individuals to the allergen; that is, they could cause a new allergy that will not show up until the next time the patient is exposed to the allergen.

Sensitivities

In a blood test, the amount of serum IgE contained within the patient's serum is measured using different immunoassays. IgG ("Type-II") allergies can be measured in blood using an enzyme-linked immunosorbent assay (ELISA) test. It is a simple blood draw, and some insurance companies will reimburse the cost. However, this type of testing is not 100% accurate, since the response will be higher to antigens currently in the diet.

For information on having your doctor or allergist order the test, contact the lab directly and request that a test kit be sent to your home or doctor's office. If the doctor is reluctant to order it, say that you are prepared to pay out of pocket if the insurance claim is rejected. Since most hospital labs are unfamiliar with

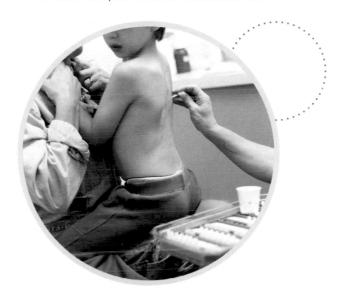

the test, instructions are included for the lab technician. You may need to wait 30 minutes for the blood to be processed and have an express delivery company pick it up from your home (at no cost to you), but many hospital labs will send it directly.

Unfortunately, there seems to be a great deal of inconsistency in the test results from every type of food allergy testing. When a sample is split and sent to several labs, or even to one lab, the results can vary widely. False negatives are the most common problem reported, which is why many doctors recommend a program of eliminating and reintroducing foods in addition to food allergy testing.

Even with these limitations, IgE allergy testing is reasonably inexpensive, and can prove to be useful. An IgG food allergy panel can be a good guideline when getting started on an elimination diet. If a food tests very high (i.e., +3 or +4), there is a good chance that your child will not tolerate it well. Keep in mind that IgG intolerances tend to subside when the food has been avoided for a period of weeks or months — so if your child is sensitive to eggs and strictly avoids them for a few months, he may be able to better tolerate them in the future (at which time rotating the food into the diet every few days is a wise policy since constant exposure is likely to increase sensitivity again).

A child with multiple intolerances is likely to have a significant problem with gut permeability, and when these values go down, it is a good sign that the gut may be beginning to heal. Retesting every 6 months is the best way to get an overall sense of what is working. The tests usually cost between $150 and $400, and the techniques can vary, so do a little research to find out which labs you think are best.

Elimination Diets

Because it is important to find out which foods cause problems for your child, many parents turn to allergy testing. However, since results are often equivocal, many people believe that an elimination diet is the most accurate way to determine what foods, if any, cause a reaction. In some cases this may be a classic allergy, and in others it may be a food intolerance. It is especially hard to determine conclusively whether or not a food is causing physical or behavioral symptoms.

An elimination diet is simple, if not always easy: Foods suspected of causing symptoms are removed from the diet, and slowly added back. For children the most common culprits are milk, wheat, eggs, peanuts, tree nuts, and soy. However, grains, vegetables, fruits, and spices may also cause problems. Often an elimination diet begins with just a few foods that are known not to provoke a reaction. Once you have taken the diet down to "bare bones," other foods are added back, one at a time, to see if they are a problem. It is important to add only one food at a time and keep a food diary. Taking careful notes will help identify any delayed reactions. Usually a food is added for one day, and then removed for a few days.

A second challenge with the same food should follow if there was no reaction, or if you are unsure about whether a delayed reaction was caused by that food. When a food's safety has been determined, another can be added in the same manner.

Some people remove only one food at a time to see if symptoms disappear, then challenge with that food. However, a regular elimination diet is often the fastest and easiest way to determine food sensitivities. Since many children on the autism spectrum eat few foods, this may be less difficult than it sounds.

Because the elimination diet is so Spartan, it is often referred to as the "cave man" diet. In general, foods allowed include lamb (preferably organic, with no chemicals or antibiotics), wild game, deep-water fish (halibut and wild-caught salmon), turkey (fresh, with no additives), vegetables (except corn and white potato) small servings of fresh, unprocessed fruit (except tomato, citrus, and fruit juice). However, lemon and lime may be used to enhance flavor. Water is the only drink given during an elimination diet. Oils used for cooking should be cold-pressed (e.g., sunflower, sesame, safflower, sesame, extra virgin olive oil). Tree nuts may be eaten if they are not treated in any way. No legumes are allowed (e.g., beans, peanuts, peas).

If a food proves to be a problem, you may want to follow up with allergy testing. However, it is important to remember that you are treating a child, not a test result. If a test is negative for eggs, but your child clearly reacts badly to them, avoid eggs. This commonsense approach will generally lead to the best balance between sensitivities and nutrition. If your child has ever had an anaphylactic reaction to a food, that food should *never* be introduced.

Recent Research on Dietary Intervention

A study published in May 2010 (see reference at end of sidebar) claims to show that a GFCF diet has no impact on behavior, sleep, or bowel patterns. This University of Rochester study claims to be the most controlled diet research in autism to date. The trial was begun in 2003 to evaluate the effects of a GFCF diet.

The study included twenty-two children between 2½ and 5½ years of age, though only fourteen of them completed the 18-week program. During the course of the study, families were to adhere to a strictly GFCF diet, as well as participate in intensive behavioral programming. The children's nutritional status was monitored throughout the study to ensure that they received adequate nutrition and enough vitamins and minerals. Subjects were also screened for iron and vitamin D deficiency, and celiac disease and wheat allergies. (One child was excluded due to testing positive for celiac disease, and one child was excluded due to an iron deficiency.)

"It would have been wonderful for children with autism and their families if we found that the GFCF diet could really help, but this small study didn't show significant benefits," said Susan Hyman, MD, associate professor of Pediatrics at Golisano

Children's Hospital at the University of Rochester Medical Center (URMC) and principal investigator of the study that was presented on May 22, 2010, at the International Meeting for Autism Research in Philadelphia. "However, the study didn't include children with significant gastrointestinal disease. It is possible those children and other specific groups might see a benefit."

A month into the diet, subjects were challenged with snacks containing either gluten, casein, both, or a placebo in randomized order. Because these proteins were disguised in food, parents could not tell which protein they were eating or whether they were actually eating a placebo. Research staff and therapy teams were also blinded to the nature of the snack. The snacks closely looked and tasted the same, so no observers could tell which was which.

Parents, teachers, and a research assistant filled out standardized surveys about the child's behavior the day before they received the snack at 2 and 24 hours after the snack. (If the child's behavior was unusual at the scheduled snack time, the snack would be post-poned until the child was back to baseline.) In addition, the parents kept a standard diary of food intake, and sleep and bowel habits. Social interaction and language were evaluated through videotaped scoring of a standardized play session with a research assistant.

No changes in attention, activity, sleep, or frequency or quality of bowel habits were reported in the study participants. No statistically significant changes were reported in any of the fourteen children.

The investigators note that this study was not designed to look at more restrictive diets or the effect of nutritional supplements on behavior. This study was designed to look only at the effects of the removal of gluten and casein from the diet of children with autism (without celiac disease) and subsequent effect of challenges with these substances in a group of children getting early intensive behavioral intervention.

Hyman said, "This is really just the tip of the iceberg. There are many possible effects of diet, including over- and under-nutrition, on behavior in children with ASD that need to be scientifically investigated so families can make informed decisions about the therapies they choose for their children." ★

Excerpted from: University of Rochester Medical Center (2010, May 20). Popular Autism Diet Does Not Demonstrate Behavioral Improvement. ScienceDaily. Retrieved from http:// www.sciencedaily.com/releases/2010/05/100519143401.htm [accessed 27 August, 2010].

When this study was published, there was an immediate outcry from the thousands of parents and physicians who have seen the benefits of the GFCF diet. Most believe that the study was flawed from the start, and could not be expected to reliably show whether or not this intervention worked. One of the best-written responses came from Autism Network for Dietary Intervention (ANDI) co-founder Karyn Seroussi. Originally asked to be on the study design team, Karyn was removed from the project when she expressed doubts about its design. Following the publication of the results, Karyn wrote to Dr. Susan Hyman to express her feelings about it.

With her permission, I include Karyn's letter in full:

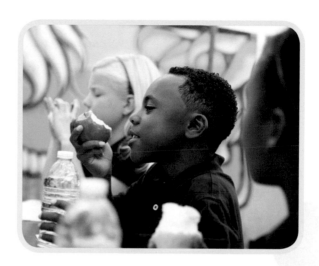

Dear Dr. Hyman,

The study results are unfortunately no surprise to me, despite the fact that I hoped I was wrong about the inherent flaws I described in 2003.

As I told you at that time, frequent challenges will almost completely nullify any hope of a positive result. The study didn't challenge children who were on a gluten- and dairy-free diet. It challenged children who were "not quite" on a gluten- and dairy-free diet. A dietary trial with a weekly challenge was as good as nothing. This study was worse than nothing, because it has now made it that much less likely that some affected children will get appropriate treatment.

According to urine tests and mountains of anecdotal evidence, it takes a couple of months before gluten and dairy peptides leave the system. Only then do challenges result in a measurable effect, and the negative effect of a provocation typically lasts about 3 weeks.

I protested about this when I was first brought in as a consultant, and was promptly removed from the team. None of the people with the most experience in dietary interventions were included in the study design. Any one of them would have told you the same thing — that the only way to examine this problem is with a matched control group and/or no challenges for at least 3 months.

The extremely small size of the study, fourteen children, bothers me considerably less than the fact that you completely ignored my input, which was given after 8 years of extensive correspondence with parents and researchers using dietary interventions.

As for the finding that there is a weak correlation between a challenge and a temporary improvement in behavior, I believe that was real, and would have been stronger if the children had actually been properly on the diet. As Jorgen and I told you when we last met, the first response to a dietary challenge is often the reverse of what one might expect: the patient becomes worse at the start of a trial, probably due to a sort of "withdrawal," and shows temporary improvement when given a new supply of opioid peptides. My stepson becomes extremely lucid after an infringement, but spends the next 3 weeks in a hyperactive stupor.

I am bewildered about how all of these resources were spent on a study that was not suitable to confirm or deny the real working hypothesis behind the diet.

~ Karyn

Dr. Robert Sears, a well-known pediatrician and author, has successfully treated many children with an autism spectrum disorder using dietary intervention. After the publication of the Hyman study, Sears published an open letter outlining his criticism (2010). Sears noted that the size of the study was too small, and the duration too short, for researchers to assess the effects of the diet accurately. He also pointed out that the study "did not remove common allergens that often play a role in autistic symptoms. Two children in the study were excluded because they tested extremely allergic to gluten. Such children would be virtually guaranteed to benefit from the diet."

An even more cynical take on this research comes from Maureen McDonnell, RN, a pediatric nurse who has treated children's health and behavioral issues using nutritional methods for 30 years. After reading the Hyman report, McDonnell (2010) shared the following response on her SOKHOP (Saving Our Kids, Healing Our Planet) website (www.sokhop.com):

Connecting the Dots

Studies have shown that many children on the autism spectrum lack the enzyme responsible for effectively breaking down gluten and casein (DPP-IV). We also know that mercury inhibits or blocks this enzyme. Now where would mercury come from? Emissions from coal-fired factories, certain large fish, amalgam dental fillings, and oh yes…many vaccines (including the flu vaccine) still contain mercury.

So if we connect the dots by looking at the facts, we see an interesting picture emerge:

1 Excess mercury blocks the enzyme that breaks down gluten and casein effectively.
2 Vaccines still contain mercury (after Uranium, the second most toxic metal on the planet).

3 Children with autism have been shown to have a difficult time excreting mercury and other toxic substances.

4 Getting rid of mercury and other toxic substances could allow the body to re-establish the enzymatic pathways that allows for the proper digestion of gluten and casein.

So here's the catch: if a study were to suggest that children with autism actually improve on a GFCF diet, it could lead one to ask why cannot they process gluten and casein in the first place? And opening that can of worms could have grave implications. This is one detective story that the pharmaceutical/vaccine industry would rather we leave unsolved.

No need for any further discussion or research on this issue: ... the diet is useless and the drugs are on their way! Ca-Ching! Ca-Ching! ★

Interestingly, another recent study came to the opposite conclusion of the Hyman research. The ScanBrit (so called because it was a collaboration between British and Scandinavian scientists) was a two-stage, 2-year randomized, controlled trial conducted in Denmark (Whitely, et al., 2010). Seventy-two subjects, children between the ages of four and ten diagnosed with autism spectrum disorders, were tested. In the first phase of the trial, the children were randomly assigned to one of two groups—an intervention group and a control group. The research team measured symptoms associated with autism using two scales (Autism Diagnostic Observation Schedule [ADOS] and Gilliam Autism Rating Scale [GARS]). The children's adaptive behaviors were assessed using the Vineland Adaptive Behavior Scales (VABS). They were also screened for symptoms of ADD and ADHD using the ADHD-IV scale.

Urine samples were collected and analyzed to see if they contained opioid peptides and/or trans-indolyl-3-acryloylglycine (IAG). The presence of these substances was a criterion for inclusion in the study since they are corre lated with a positive response to a GFCF diet. Researchers reported that the treatment group showed significant improvement at the end of the first phase of the trial. In the second phase, the treatment and control groups were combined, with all subjects following a GFCF diet. "Introducing a GFCF diet had a signifi-cant beneficial group effect at 8, 12, and 24 months of intervention on core autistic and related behaviors of prepubescent children diagnosed with ASD and pathological urinary results. The results showed a less dramatic change in group scores between 8 and 24 months, possibly reflective of a plateau effect during this period." In short, unlike the Hyman study, the ScanBrit concluded that

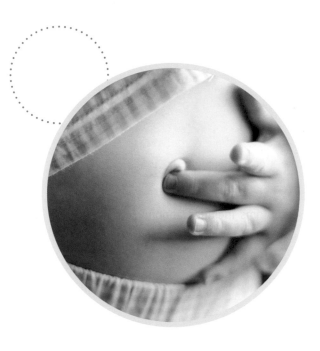

dietary intervention may have a positive effect on some children with autism.

There are also other, smaller studies that have shown support for dietary intervention. Because autism has been linked to gut pain and diarrhea, Jeremy Nicholson at Imperial College London (Geddes, 2010) studied thirty-nine children with autism, along with twenty-eight of their typical siblings and thirty-four unrelated children. Using nuclear magnetic resonance spectroscopy (NMR) to examine urine samples, the researchers found that each of these groups had a distinct chemical composition, with significant differences between children on the autism spectrum and typical controls. "The signature that comes up is related to gut bacteria," said Nicholson. They have not proven that the bacteria's metabolic products contribute to the development of autism, but Nicholson believes this is a possibility that merits further research.

Dr. Derrick MacFabe (2010) and others at the University of Western Ontario agree. Their own research showed that short-chain fatty acids produced by clostridium bacteria could induce behavioral and biochemical changes, which are associated with autism, in rats. MacFabe believes that "Nicholson's study did find some biomarkers of gut clostridial populations that we think contribute to autistic symptoms."

Research by Dr. H. Jyonouchi (Jyonouchi, et al., 2005) of the Autism Center at the University of Medical and Dentistry of New Jersey found that, relative to controls, children on the autism spectrum have an abnormal response to cow's milk protein, wheat protein, and soy protein. The reaction was strongest to milk, and in many cases, the reaction to soy was more pronounced than the reaction to wheat.

Dr. Timothy Buie, a pediatric gastroenterologist at Harvard's Mass General Hospital, has performed endoscopies with biopsies on many children with autism. He noted that there was a frequent presence of inflammation of the digestive tract (Buie, Winter & Kushak, 2002). He found that 55% of the children with autism he scoped showed abnormal levels of digestive enzymes, and concluded that they were more likely to suffer from impaired starch metabolism, carbohydrate malabsorption, and bowel disorders than typical peers. According to Buie, "These children are ill, and they are in distress and pain. They are not just mentally, neurologically dysfunctional."

Dr. Ted Kniker (2001) of the San Antonio Autistic Treatment Center in Texas, Dr. Anne-Marie Knivsberg (2002) of the Stavanger University College in Norway, Dr. S. Lucarelli (Lucarelli, et al., 1995) at the University of Rome, and other researchers have all published studies showing that some children and adults with autism improve after eliminating dairy and wheat foods from their diets. Even if we cannot be positive of the cause right now, we know that many of these children get better on special diets. Dr. Aristo Vojdani (2004) showed an increased immune response to dietary peptides in subjects who have autism, a finding that also underscores the need to remove gluten and casein from the diet.

Laura De Magistris studied gut permeability in individuals with autism and their first-degree relatives (de Magistris, et al., 2010). They found that intestinal permeability was abnormal in a significant number of the subjects and their relatives. Those who were on a GFCF diet had significantly lower intestinal permeability. They concluded that the leaky gut hypothesis was supported and that testing for intestinal permeability might identify the subgroup of children with autism who might benefit from dietary intervention.

Children with autism have only rarely been tested for gastrointestinal disorders, even when they show symptoms of common GI diseases. This may be changing, however. The Autism Speaks Autism Treatment Network recently reported on data from fifteen treatment and research centers in the United States and Canada on the relationship between GI symptoms and spectrum disorders. The study included over one thousand children diagnosed with autism, pervasive developmental disorder (PDD), or Asperger's Syndrome. The study showed that 45% of the children had GI symptoms at the time of enrollment. These symptoms included abdominal pain, constipation, and diarrhea. "These findings suggest that better evaluation of GI symptoms and subsequent treatment may have benefits for these patients," according to Dr. Daniel Coury (Blazek, 2010), the medical director of

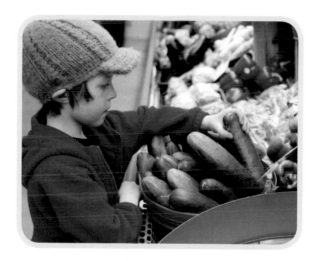

the Autism Treatment Network and professor of pediatrics and psychiatry at Ohio State University.

Sadly, children who were tested and found to suffer from GI disorders were excluded from the Rochester study. (See sidebar at beginning of this chapter.) Since these are the very children who might be expected to benefit the most from a special diet, it is bewildering to ponder this exclusion.

In addition to removing problematic proteins from the diet, dietary intervention for our children (not just the ones with spectrum disorders) should include the following:

- Improve the quality of the diet, reducing sugars, additives, and toxins from pesticides.
- Identify food allergies and sensitivities and remove offending foods.
- Identify and correct nutritional deficiencies with appropriate supplements.
- Diagnose and treat gastrointestinal illnesses or disorders.
- Use probiotic foods and supplements, as well as antifungal or antibacterial medicines, to correct dysbiosis.

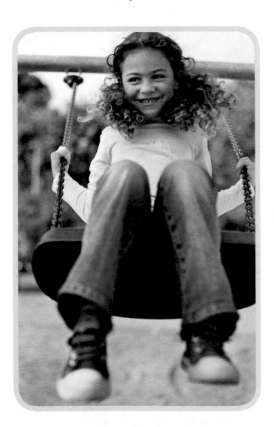

Other Dietary Issues in Autism

Avoiding gluten, and a similar dairy protein called casein, is at the heart of the dietary intervention outlined in this book. Unfortunately, many children seem to need dietary modifications that go beyond simply avoiding gluten and casein. Many children must also avoid soy, corn, and eggs. Some are on a restricted carbohydrate diet such as the **Specific Carbohydrate Diet (SCD)** or Body Ecology Diet **(BED)**. Some children are now on the Low Oxalate Diet **(LOD)**, a diet that limits oxalates found in many foods. Most must limit sugar and increase fermented and other probiotic foods.

Specific Carbohydrate Diet (SCD)

The Specific Carbohydrate Diet is a special type of GF diet, developed by Dr. Sidney Valentine Haas (1951), described in the book *The Management of Celiac Disease*. Originally developed to treat Crohn's disease, ulcerative colitis, celiac disease, and cystic fibrosis, the SCD has also been used successfully for treating "failure to thrive," severe diarrhea, and other gastrointestinal problems.

After her daughter responded to this diet, the late Elaine Gottschall wrote a groundbreaking book on the topic called *Breaking the Vicious Cycle: Intestinal Health Through Diet*. This book inspired many families to find out whether the SCD could be helpful for their children who have autism.

This diet is based on the premise that damaged intestinal walls and bacterial overgrowth from undigested carbohydrates cause immune dysfunction and poor health. Because the bacteria are believed to feed on these complex sugars and starches, restricting them should restore the proper ecology of intestinal flora and allow the gut to heal. Reducing the immune load on the gut may also greatly reduce food sensitivities; after a year on the diet, some people report that their intolerances have been reduced or resolved. Many children with a history of gastrointestinal problems have greatly benefited from the SCD.

The SCD is simple, though not easy (at least at first). The diet is limited to monosaccharides. These are the simplest form of carbohydrate, consisting of one molecule of sugar. These require minimal digestion and are easily absorbed. That means that the SCD, which eliminates all starches and most sugars, consists mainly of meats, fish, eggs, vegetables, fruits, nuts, and seeds. (For a list of "safe foods" visit www.breakingthevicious-cycle.info). Other potentially problematic foods, such as chocolate and soy, are also removed. Although some types of dairy are allowed on the original version of this diet, casein tends to remain a problem for children on the autism spectrum, so many families opt to do a non-dairy version of the SCD.

There are many children who make only minor improvement on a GFCF diet, despite strict adherence. Proponents of the SCD suggest that these children cannot implant normal flora, even with careful supplementation. They may also continue to show deficiencies in vitamins, minerals, fatty acids, and amino acids. Therefore, those on a GFCF diet who continue to have chronic yeast overgrowth, *Clostridia*, gas, bloating, diarrhea, or constipation are good candidates for the SCD.

For GI disorders, such as ulcerative colitis and Crohn's Disease, strict adherence to the SCD is required for healing and the relief of symptoms. SCD proponents say that the same rigorous adherence is necessary to achieve full results in the case of children with autism.

Some parents have noted that cutting out a substantial amount of starches and sugars will yield significant benefits, and that the level of adherence can be fine-tuned to meet the needs of the individual and the family. However, it is difficult to say how much is "too much," and words like *limit, restrict,* and *reduce* can mean different things to different people. A big advantage of the SCD is that its guidelines are an absolute: *monosaccharides only.*

Therefore, if you have decided to reduce the amount of starch and sugar in your child's diet, it makes sense to start with a trial on the SCD, which is bound to help break your child's addiction to these foods. Follow the guidelines specially designed for ASD children at www.pecanbread.com, and ask for support from experienced parents. Even if you see a pattern of ill health that does not improve and you decide to try a different diet, your child will probably be eating nutritious foods that you never dreamed would cross his lips.

As with other special diets, a regression may occur at the start. It is important to not become discouraged. Some people recommend a gradual removal of complex carbohydrates and sugars to reduce the severity of a die-off reaction.

The SCD is divided into stages, with the first stage consisting of easily digested foods. As the gut heals and inflammation of the tissue is reduced, more foods are introduced. The SCD only allows beans after there has been some gut healing, and then, only if there are no negative reactions. It is important to follow the SCD guidelines for introductions

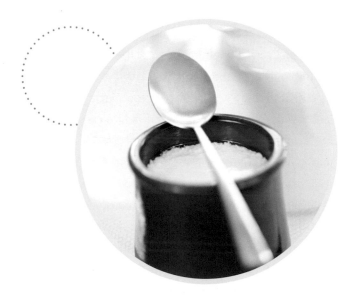

of foods, and not proceed too quickly. For example, even if you decide to try a specially prepared goat yogurt, you should not do so for at least a month. While digestive enzymes are not required, many have found that they make the SCD more effective.

The SCD is widely supported by the autism community, and talks on this diet are included in the Defeat Autism Now! Conferences. In addition to the thousands of children following a strict SCD, there are countless others on a modified version, which could be referred to as a "Restricted Carbohydrate Diet." These modifications may stray from the original principles laid down by Dr. Haas, but when the elimination of complex sugars is the primary principle of a diet, it is widely referred to as the SCD.

Many children suffer from an increased yeast overgrowth at the outset of the SCD because bacterial pathogens are the first to die, leaving room for yeast to grow. Since yeast feeds on starches and sugars, it is best to limit the intake of honey and fruits initially. It is also helpful to lightly cook fruits, causing the breakdown of natural sugars prior to ingestion. Pathogenic bacteria can cause the symptoms of fructose malabsorption, so once the dysbiosis has been addressed, fruit may be slowly added back into the diet.

Some children experience a worsening of constipation when the diet is first started. Pecanbread.com provides a protocol for addressing this. Another concern is that those with oxalate issues may react poorly if they are eating a significant number of almonds or other tree nuts.

A specially prepared goat yogurt is the preferred way to provide probiotics; advocates maintain that after some healing has occurred, the goat yogurt may be tolerated even by those who were sensitive to casein. If a child has a milk allergy, or a parent prefers not to use any dairy products, nut yogurts and other fermented foods can be used.

A great deal of support and information is available at Pecanbread.com. There are also online discussion groups and lists to provide parent-to-parent support such as http://health.groups.yahoo.com/group/pecanbread.

Restricted Carbohydrate Diets for Children with Multiple Food Allergies

One concern that many parents have when implementing this diet is that children with peanut, tree nut, and egg allergies may have trouble getting adequate nutrition from a wide variety of foods. There is now a special web page with instructions for gaining weight and for tracking the caloric content of the child's diet to insure that the child gets an adequate amount of calories; it can be found in the "Overcoming Difficulties" section of the Pecanbread.com.

Although there have been many SCD success stories, there are also children who require modifications to a strictly starch-free regimen. It is difficult to know when to persist with a special diet and when to change course, which is why it is so important to get support from those who are experienced with this diet and to have your child under the supervision of a qualified nutritionist.

The Body Ecology Diet (BED)

The Body Ecology Diet is a dietary program targeting fungal infections, viruses, and parasites. It promotes health and healing using high quality, easily digested foods plentiful in healthy fats and minerals. The diet draws from the principles of several other types of diets, including macrobiotics, raw foods, blood type, Weston A. Price, and the Yeast Connection. In 2003, the diet began to receive interest from the autism community since unhealthy flora is linked with food allergies and GI dysfunction.

The premise of the diet is that many cases of chronic illness begin with a fungal infection in the gut. The gut becomes unable to perform its job as the first line of defense for the immune system, which leads to various secondary illnesses. Incompletely digested nutrients inside the gut wall lead to allergic reactions, and nutrients are improperly absorbed, leading to nutritional deficiency. If these pathogenic organisms escape the intestines, they can provoke symptoms affecting the rest of the body.

The solution, then, is to first heal the gut by re-establishing the correct gut flora, and then nourish and rebuild the body. The BED is designed to do those things, based on the following principles:

1 **The Expansion/Contraction Principle:** This is a principle from macrobiotics that looks at the "energetic" properties of food. Certain foods are seen as "contracting" such as meat, eggs, and salt. Other foods are seen as "expanding" such as sugars. The BED encourages primary food selection from the middle of this continuum, emphasizing lots of vegetables.

2 **The Acid/Alkaline Principle:** This is a commonly used principle in alternative medicine/nutrition. It is based on the idea

that the blood should be kept slightly alkaline, which is thought to discourage candidiasis and the growth and spread of cancer. It is suggested that every meal contain 20% "acid-forming" foods and 80% "alkaline-forming" foods.

3 The Uniqueness Principle: This principle acknowledges that one size does not fit all in diets. For example, some people may do better with a slightly higher percentage of protein in their diet, and some people may tolerate animal protein better than others. Each person is encouraged to respect the signals that their body sends, and to avoid foods that do not work for them.

4 The Cleansing Principle: This principle states that we must be continually cleansing to attain and maintain good health. Modern-day living is full of exposures to toxins, and these toxins must be continuously removed. Regular bowel cleansing is recommended to assist with this process.

5 The Food Combining Principle: The basic premise is that different macronutrients need different conditions in the stomach to be properly digested. For example, protein requires a high-acid environment. Starch, on the other hand, requires a more alkaline environment to digest properly. If you mix starch and protein in a single meal, the stomach cannot properly set the conditions to digest, so it cannot do a good job with either component. By eating fruit separately, and separating starch and protein into separate meals, you increase the efficiency of digestion and reduce unwanted fermentation. (It has been suggested that this is a good way to start the diet for sensitive children, and then move on to the other principles.)

6 The 80/20 Principle: This principle is taken from Oriental medicine, which states that you should never eat more than 80% of your stomach capacity in one meal. This leaves you with 20% of your stomach empty, giving it room to properly mix the meal with enzymes and acid.

7 The Step by Step Principle: This principle states that healing comes in steps, which happen in their own time and order. When people are really sick, they may not have the capacity to handle a full-blown "healing crisis." So the body will go through cycles of progress followed by a rest period. Each step reaches deeper into the body to pull out toxins and heal the affected organs.

By healing the gut, re-establishing the healthy microflora, and providing the body with nutritious foods, the body is then able to build itself up to the point that it can begin to detoxify. The liver is able to do its job of removing the toxins from the body. The gut will allow the nutrients through to feed the brain, thyroid, and adrenals to begin detoxifying and healing. The BED has also been suggested for the mothers of the children with autism, as they may also suffer from fungal infections and complaints of fibromyalgia, chronic fatigue, and eczema.

The BED is a GF diet focusing on the use of minimally processed, healthy foods. It consists of large amounts of vegetables (including sea vegetables), meats, eggs, good fats,

Celtic sea salt, and herbs for seasoning. The grains recommended in the BED are quinoa, amaranth, buckwheat, and millet. All of these grains are gluten-free, and said to "alkalinize" the body. The BED also recommends certain therapeutic foods, which are specifically aimed at re-establishing the intestinal flora and healing the body. Those on the diet must daily eat and drink foods that are fermented or cultured.

If you decide to try the BED, do so with the support of experienced people who have been using the diet for several months or years, and under the supervision of a qualified medical professional. Details can be found in the book, *The Body Ecology Diet*, by Donna Gates. Additional information, including products helpful in implementing the diet, can be found at www.bodyecologydiet.com. For online information about the BED and children with autism, and to join a support group/message board, go to www.bedrokcommunity.org. For BED support for adults and teens, try http://health.groups.yahoo.com/group/beginnerBEDROK/.

Low Oxalate Diet (LOD)

Oxalates are tiny salts found in some plant foods. Moderate amounts are not harmful for healthy individuals, but have been known to create problems for those with certain health conditions (e.g., kidney stones), in conditions where there is a loss of gut integrity (e.g., gastric bypass surgery), some types of bowel disease (e.g., Crohn's, celiac), and in cystic fibrosis.

Autism researcher Susan Owens (2005) suggested the LOD for children with autism because of the leaky gut and gut inflammation often seen in children who have autism. She pointed out that oxalates from food in a healthy gut should pass through the body harmlessly bound to minerals like calcium, or else degraded ("eaten") by protective gut bacteria like *Oxalobacter formigenes*. If these minerals or microflora are deficient, unbound oxalate can be absorbed in the intestines,

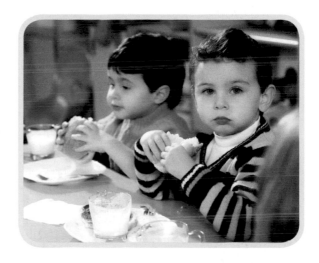

where it will travel through the gaps between cells and into the blood. From there, oxalates will end up in tissues of the body, worsening pain and inflammation throughout, and impairing many enzymes involved in energy metabolism and defense against yeast and dysbiosis. Oxalates can worsen sulfation issues, and greatly increase oxidative stress. Oxalates may be part of the reason why a host of problems arise from immune dysfunction, allergies, imbalanced microflora, mineral deficiency, and increased intestinal permeability.

Foods high in oxalates should not be a problem for most healthy people. However, without certain minerals or the right sort of bacteria, the unbound oxalate can slip through gaps in a leaky gut and cause inflammation throughout the body. Oxalates from

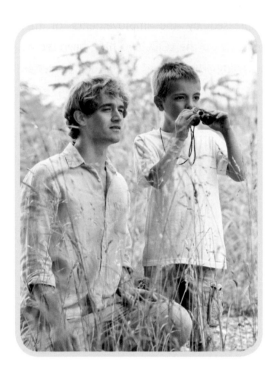

food, or that are secreted by the body, may also keep the gut from healing properly. Therefore, sharply reducing oxalates in the diet could speed up the process of healing a damaged gut. Some parents have had success combining principles from the Low Oxalate Diet and the Specific Carbohydrate Diet, or Body Ecology Diet, to promote the fastest healing for inflamed tissue.

Children who have done poorly on special diets based on nuts, or on grains and certain vegetables, are likely candidates for success

on the LOD, as well as those who have steatorrhea (fat in the stool) or poor function of the upper intestine. Those with urinary issues, pain or stiffness, low energy, poor growth, or skin issues that will not resolve may also benefit. Gluten-containing foods are often high in oxalates, which may explain why some people suffering from these symptoms find that they improve on a GF diet. Owens encourages those on LOD to stay or become gluten-free, since gluten may have the effect of increasing gut permeability.

Testing for high oxalates is now being offered on some organic acids tests. However, initial clinical data suggests that urine testing is not predictive of success on this diet — some of the best responders are patients who had very low levels of oxalate in their urine before starting the LOD. This may be due to a problem in the kidney's ability to excrete oxalate, stemming from the sulfation problems common in persons with autism.

Owens advises starting the diet by first cutting back the very high-oxalate foods, then slowly moving to lower oxalate foods, one food at a time, until the oxalate count is below 40 milligrams for /2,000 calories per day. *The Low Oxalate Cookbook, Version II** contains extensive information on oxalate content per serving, and you can find a comprehensive food list with oxalate content and other food traits at www.lowoxalate.info/recipes.html. As with many autism treatments, an early worsening may be seen as a good sign, but if the negative symptoms are severe, you should decrease the rate at which you are lowering oxalates and use some recommended supplements. After the "detox process" is finished, which can take from a couple of months to a couple of years, then high-oxalate foods can be cautiously added back into the diet one by one.

Progress on the LOD usually occurs only after the body starts the cyclic process of freeing up oxalate from tissues. Those who had previously been eating a high-oxalate diet are most likely to suffer from a regression in the first stages of the diet as built-up oxalates are released from the body. This usually involves some obvious negative symptoms after a few days such as diarrhea, urinary discomfort, behavioral changes, upper respiratory congestion, or skin rashes. Parents sometimes refer to this as the "dump."

If this diet is helpful, you should notice (between "dumps") improvements in the areas of physical comfort, complex thinking, sociability, speech, gross and fine motor skills, energy, loss of stiffness, and skin problems such as eczema. Your child may be willing to eat foods he avoided before, and may stop craving high- oxalate foods. He or she may have an increase in appetite. A child with delayed growth may suddenly have a growth spurt. However, if there is no change for the better or worse after 2 weeks on a very low-oxalate diet, assuming that the guidelines for supplements are being followed, then this diet will probably not be helpful.

Although it may be necessary to continue to restrict foods that are very high in oxalates, this diet is not meant to be a lifetime program

for the treatment of autism. After some time on the LOD, when healing has taken place and symptoms of ill health have improved, it should be possible to increase the amount of oxalate in the diet without ill effects.

Although initially skeptical about "yet another diet," many physicians have been impressed by the improvements of their patients on the LOD, and have been recommending a trial period on the diet for certain individuals with inflammation and/or GI symptoms. There are over two thousand members in the "Trying Low Oxalates" online support group.

During the "dumping" period, one may notice a temporary worsening or onset of urinary issues such as penis pain or redness, urinary frequency, or urinary urgency. There might be unusual skin rashes, including *livedo reticularis*, which is an inflammation of blood vessels that makes them show up vividly in the skin like a road map. Oxalate crystals can

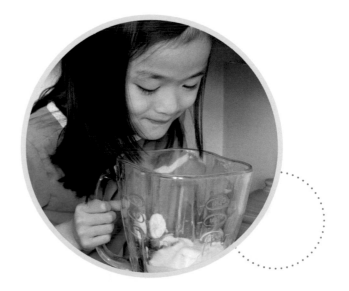

cause gum problems, so if teeth begin to feel loose, one should slow down and increase antioxidant protection. There might also be an onset of diarrhea, including sandy stools and stools with black specks.

In some children, previous infections may reappear (e.g., streptococcus, Pediatric Auto-immune Neuropsychiatric Disorders Associated with Streptococcal infection [PANDAS]). Why this happens is unknown, but it has

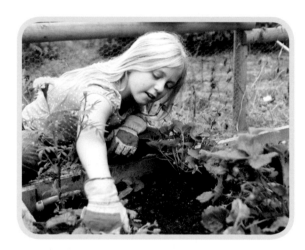

been theorized that some of the bacteria was trapped by oxalate crystals and later liberated when the crystals broke down.

Keep in mind that these "dumping" symptoms should not show up in someone unless they have had an oxalate problem. These bad periods tend to be followed by resolution of earlier symptoms, as well as global improvements.

A further concern is that some people are prone to constipation on the LOD, possibly a result of the reduced amount of fiber from vegetables and whole grains. Calcium supplements (see page 40) can also be constipating

to those who are sensitive to them. Owens suggests trying different types of calcium, switching to magnesium citrate, or using a combination of the two (magnesium tends to be helpful for constipation—you can adjust the proportions until you hit the right balance). Ground flax seeds are relatively low in oxalates compared to other seeds; they are a good source of fiber and may be helpful in treating constipation.

High doses of probiotic supplements or cultured foods are recommended before starting this diet because they can help degrade oxalates. Total intake of vitamin C should not exceed 250 milligrams per day because it can worsen an oxalate problem in the body. It was once thought that calcium was also problematic; however, studies have shown it is important to provide enough calcium orally (preferably calcium citrate) to bind to the free oxalate in the gut and form calcium oxalate, which can pass through the body without being absorbed. This should be taken without vitamin D about 10 minutes before meals.

Other supplements are recommended for the LOD, or should be avoided, so read through the guidelines at www.lowoxalate.info/faqs.html. To get support for this diet, and to see lists of high- and low-oxalate foods, join the online support group at www.yahoogroups.com/group/Trying_Low_Oxalates.

*The Vulvar Pain Foundation has published two excellent cookbooks filled with low-oxalate recipes, and comprehensive lists of food oxalate levels. You can order them from Wellnesshealth.com, or check out www.vulvarpainfoundation.org, telephone: (336) 226-0704.

Because it can be confusing, most people referring to any of these interventions just say **GFCF diet**. Since experience has shown that most people on the autism spectrum will benefit from a diet free of gluten and casein, the removal of these foods should be considered the foundation for dietary intervention. Because our children are all unique, it makes sense to start there and then tweak until we get it right.

If we focus on the biological basis of autism spectrum disorders, a pattern emerges:

- A child may be genetically predisposed to improper immune response.
- Some "load" triggers abnormal immune response. This load may be vaccines, or some component of vaccines, or it may be another environmental factor.
- The child is frequently ill due to decreased immunity.
- Antibiotics are given (though infections are often viral).
- "Good" gut flora are wiped out because of antibiotic use and/or by the impairment in the immune system; *Candida* (yeast) overgrowth causes gut damage.
- Mercury in vaccines may inhibit enzymes needed to break down peptides.
- An inability to process certain proteins, such as gluten and casein, develops, perhaps because of enzyme deficiency.
- Improperly digested peptides escape the damaged gut into the bloodstream.
- Opioid peptides mimic neurotransmitters and scramble signals.

Mounting evidence suggests that the dietary interventions described in this book are potentially helpful for a wide range of diseases and disorders—especially for a growing part of our population: those with autism spectrum disorder. As unlikely as it may seem, dietary intervention can really help some children with autism by removing biologically active peptides and allergens, thus reducing the load on an over-taxed detoxification system. Everyone has heard the old saying, "You are what you eat." However, it is probably more accurate to say, "You are what you digest!"

Testing and Nutritional Support

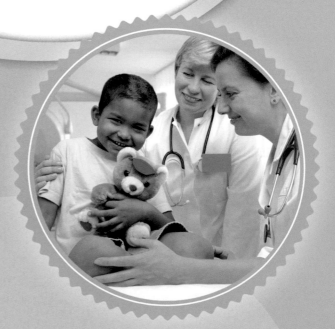

When parents first begin biomedical intervention, a vast number of blood and urine tests may be recommended. The array of tests available is confusing, and determining which tests are most likely to identify treatable problems for individuals on the autism spectrum can be difficult. Running every test available may be too expensive (many are not covered by insurance) and may not produce significant information. If resources are limited, ask your doctor to limit the prescribed tests to those that can provide treatment options (rather than tests that merely add to the doctor's knowledge or research).

In other words, you may want to prioritize the tests with your doctor, based on likely benefit and cost. Whenever possible, do testing prior to starting dietary intervention since removal of gluten could affect the outcome of the test;

a celiac who is on a gluten-free diet may have a negative test result.

The following are tests recommended by Sidney Baker, MD, (1997), and Jon Pangborn, Ph.D., (2008) co-founders of Defeat Autism

Now! Detailed information about understanding and interpreting the results of these tests can be found in their book, *Autism: Effective Biomedical Treatments*.

- Blood Chemistry and CBC Analysis
- Comprehensive Stool Analysis
- Ammonia
- Genetic Testing
- Intestinal Permeability
- Celiac Disease
- Allergy Testing for Food/Inhalants
- Organic Acids Analysis
- Fatty Acids Analysis
- Element Analysis and Metallothionein Assessments
- Immune Testing
- Urinary Peptide Analysis
- Toxic Levels of Mercury and other Heavy Metals

In addition, make sure your doctor helps you identify and address any nutritional deficiencies, and follow up with further tests if necessary.

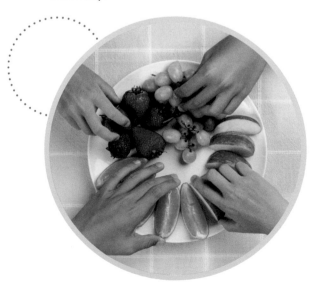

If your child becomes upset over blood draws, ask your doctor to prescribe EMLA Cream before the testing day. This cream numbs the skin so that a needle stick is painless. Slather some on both of his inner arms about 1 hour before your appointment and wrap some plastic wrap loosely around them to keep from wiping off before the blood draw.

Vitamins and Minerals

Children on the autism spectrum rarely eat a balanced diet. Even those who are not on a restricted diet typically eat a narrow range of foods. The fact that these children need dietary supplements has been confirmed by double-blind, placebo-controlled studies. One study found that a strong, balanced multivitamin/mineral supplement resulted in improvements in children with autism in sleep and gut function, and possibly in other areas.

When you further restrict the diets, for example by removing dairy, then you must also add calcium, magnesium and vitamin D from other food sources, usually from supplements. Children on the autism spectrum may need to take more supplements than a typical child. Your doctor will want to run blood tests to measure vitamin and mineral levels and look for other deficiencies. Some may need to take B vitamins in doses above the RDA (recommended daily allowance).

Vitamins are nutrients we need to stay alive. They are essential for our bodies to function normally and many must be supplied because the body does not make them. Along with other nutrients (proteins, fats, carbohydrates, and minerals), they are required for children to grow and for all humans to live. All the essential vitamins must be supplied by the diet or supplemented for a person to be healthy. Please keep in mind that you should not exceed the recommended maximum dose of any vitamin unless your doctor has determined that this is appropriate for your child.

Vitamins that May Be Deficient in Those with Autism Spectrum Disorder

Vitamin A is a fat-soluble nutrient; it is often called beta-carotene on food labels. Vitamin A exists in two forms, retinol and carotene. Retinol is found only in foods of animal origin. Carotene can be found in both animal and plant foods. Beta-carotene is the most common form found in multivitamins. Vitamin A is important for eye health and builds resistance to respiratory infections. Non-dairy food sources include egg yolks, sweet potatoes, winter squash, and cantaloupe. Vitamin A works best when taken with B complex, vitamin D, vitamin E, calcium, phosphorus, and zinc.

Vitamin B_1 is also called thiamine. It is water-soluble, so any excess is excreted. Thiamine promotes normal appetite and aids digestion (especially of carbohydrates). It should be taken with other B vitamins. For children on restricted diets, there are not many appropriate foods sources other than legumes and peanuts. This vitamin is destroyed by heat and oxidation.

Vitamin B_2 is also called riboflavin. It is not destroyed by heat but by light (especially ultraviolet light). Riboflavin is important for growth and healthy skin, hair, and nails. Food sources include leafy green vegetables and fish.

Vitamin B_5 is also called pantothenic acid. It can be made in the body. It is important for the function of the adrenal glands,

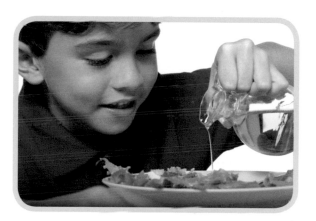

and needed for the conversion of fat and sugar to energy. It is needed to make infection-fighting antibodies. Dietary sources include meats, egg yolks, peanuts, chicken, and green vegetables.

Vitamin B_6 is also called pyridoxine. This vitamin is needed for the production of red blood cells and antibodies. It is essential for the proper absorption of other B vitamins. B_6 is actually a group of nutrients (pyridoxine, pyridoxinal, and pyridoxamine) that function together and are required for the production of some digestive enzymes and protein metabolism. B_6 is important for the nervous system, and helps to assimilate protein and fat. Most of the multivitamins formulated for children on the autism spectrum include fairly large doses of B_6. Dietary sources include meat, poultry, fish, shellfish, cabbage, and cantaloupe.

In persons with autism, it has been reported that B_6 is most effective when taken with magnesium, which will usually counteract any hyperactivity that arises from the B_6. According to more than five thousand parent responses on the ARI Treatment Checklist, nearly one-half of patients with autism benefit from the combination of B_6 plus magnesium.

Vitamin B_{12} is also called cobalamin. Important for growth, concentration, memory, and balance, cobalamin also forms and regenerates red blood cells. It is important for a healthy nervous system. It can be found in

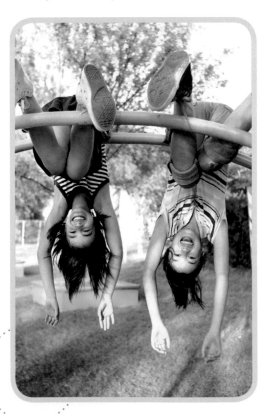

beef, pork, fish, shellfish, and eggs. In 2002 James Neubrander, a Defeat Autism Now! doctor, made the discovery that the type of B_{12} called methyl-cobalamin was very helpful to children on the autism spectrum; methyl-cobalamin is closely allied with the folic acid biochemical pathway and is necessary for detoxification (James, et al., 2004). For children who have autism and a deficiency in this enzyme, supplementing with methyl-cobalamin improves detoxification. The most effective method of administration is by injection, using a very thin needle tolerated well by most children. Compounding pharmacists are able to preload the single-dose syringes, and parents inject their children on a schedule determined by their doctor. Dr. Neubrander and others have reported huge gains in language, socialization, and behavior when this procedure is used.

Biotin is another member of the B-complex family of vitamins. It is important for metabolism. It is said to help alleviate eczema and other skin problems. Dietary biotin can be found in egg yolks, unpolished rice, almonds, walnuts, and fruits. Biotin is one of the few vitamins that can be synthesized in the body by intestinal bacteria.

Choline and inositol are B-complex members that work together to use fats and cholesterol. Combined they form lecithin. Choline is one of the few substances known to cross the blood-brain barrier. It helps memory, has a soothing effect, and assists in detoxification. Dietary sources include egg yolks and green leafy vegetables. Wheat is one of the main sources, so children using any dietary intervention may be deficient. Most multivitamins contain approximately 50 milligrams of choline and inositol; these two nutrients are always kept in balance.

Vitamin C is also called ascorbic acid. This water-soluble vitamin is usually supplied by citrus fruits and juices, but it is also in strawberries, green and leafy vegetables, potatoes, sweet potatoes, and cantaloupe. It is important in the formation of collagen, a component of bones and cartilage, and for the absorption of iron. A potent antioxidant, vitamin C is said to help prevent viral and bacterial infections, and reduce the effects of some allergens. For those reducing oxalates, vitamin C should be limited to no more than 250 milligrams per day.

Vitamin D is also called calciferol. It is a fat-soluble vitamin normally acquired through diet and exposure to sunlight. Vitamin D promotes strong bones and teeth by enabling the proper absorption of calcium and phosphorus (this is why milk is usually fortified with vitamin D). Non-dairy sources include salmon, tuna, egg yolks, fish oils, and oily fish such as sardines and herring. Most people in northern climates, especially those with medium to dark skin, do not get sufficient vitamin D from sunlight. However, even in sunny climates, some people may be chronically deficient. Doctors report that low levels of vitamin D are almost universal in their patients, which means that they are not benefiting from the considerable anti-inflammatory properties of this vitamin. A

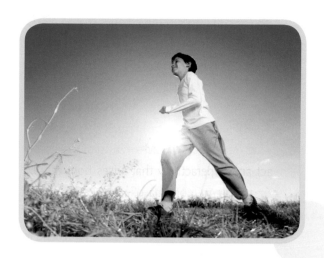

childhood deficiency of vitamin D has also been linked with the onset of multiple sclerosis in adulthood, further emphasizing the need for adequate supplementation.

Vitamin E is also called tocopherol. Unlike other fat-soluble vitamins, very little vitamin E is stored in the body, with approximately 65% of the daily dose being excreted in the stool. Vitamin E is an important antioxidant, preventing oxidation of fat compounds, vitamins A and C, and some amino acids. It is important for healing and to prevent cell damage. Dietary sources include vegetable oils, broccoli, Brussels sprouts, eggs, spinach, and soybeans.

Folates and folic acid are forms of water-soluble B vitamins. Folic acid refers to the synthetic vitamin used in supplements, while folates, including folinic acid, are the form found in foods. Folates are critical for the proper development and maintenance of cells, especially during times of rapid cell division such as fetal development and childhood. It was discovered several years ago to be critically important for preventing neural tube birth defects, and pregnant women were advised to take a daily supplement of folic acid. Folate deficiency is believed to be the most common vitamin deficiency in the world due to food processing, food selection, and intestinal disorders. People with food sensitivities and environmental illnesses who are deficient in B vitamins may see some clear improvements from supplementation.

Minerals that May Be Deficient in Those with Autism Disorders

Calcium works with phosphorus to build healthy bones and teeth. It also helps the body use iron, helps nutrients pass through cell walls, keeps the heart beating regularly, and metabolizes iron. There must be sufficient vitamin D for calcium to be absorbed. Proper absorption of calcium can be inhibited by large amounts of fat, oxalic acid. Those on dairy-free diets need to monitor their overall

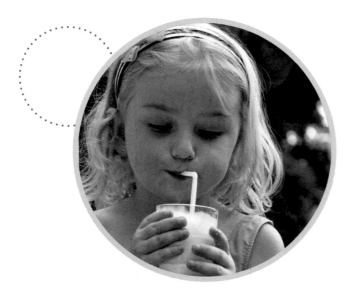

calcium intake. **Note:** Calcium can cause or worsen constipation. Adequate doses of magnesium may counteract that effect.

Copper is required for converting iron into hemoglobin. It is also important for the utilization of vitamin C. However, too much copper can cause sleep disturbances and other problems. Dr. William Walsh of the Walsh Research Institute reports that the test results of children on the autism spectrum typically show abnormalities in the ratio of copper to zinc, which can be corrected with supplementation.

Iron is a critically important mineral, essential for the production of hemoglobin, myoglobin (red pigment in muscles), and some enzymes. It is also important for the metabolism of the various B vitamins. Iron is important for growth and prevents anemia and fatigue. The best dietary sources are meat, clams, egg yolks, cashews, hazelnuts, and molasses.

Magnesium is sometimes called the serenity mineral because it can be calming and improves mood and appetite. In many cases, it can help relieve or reduce constipation. Magnesium is required for calcium and vitamin C metabolism and is essential for nerve and muscle function. Dietary sources include squash, fish, figs, grapefruit, lemons, corn, almonds, seeds, and dark green vegetables. It has been reported that magnesium is most effective for those with autism when taken with vitamin B_6.

Phosphorus is involved in every physiological chemical reaction. It is needed for normal heart and kidney function. It is found in fish, poultry, meat, eggs, tree nuts, peanuts, and seeds. Calcium and vitamin D are necessary for proper phosphorus function.

Zinc is often found to be low in children on the autism spectrum (with corresponding high levels of copper). Zinc is an important mineral, involved in the maintenance of enzyme systems. It helps form insulin and is essential for protein metabolism. It helps maintain the acid-alkaline balance and is important to brain function. It promotes growth and increases mental alertness. Because it naturally stimulates appetite, some doctors recommend zinc supplementation when a child will not eat enough. Although there are many dietary sources of zinc, most of it is destroyed in processing. Many plants are also lower in zinc than previously thought because of soil that has been depleted of nutrients.

Some signs of zinc deficiency are impairment of taste, a poor immune response, and skin problems. Other symptoms of zinc deficiency can include hair loss, diarrhea, fatigue, delayed wound healing, and decreased growth rate and mental development in infants. It is thought that zinc supplementation can help skin conditions, such as acne and eczema, prostate problems, and anorexia nervosa. White spots on the fingernails can also indicate a zinc deficiency. Zinc is highly recommended for those on the autism spectrum and their families. According to Dr. Sidney Baker the serum zinc level in his patients with autism is usually marginal or sub-normal.

How and What to Feed Your Child

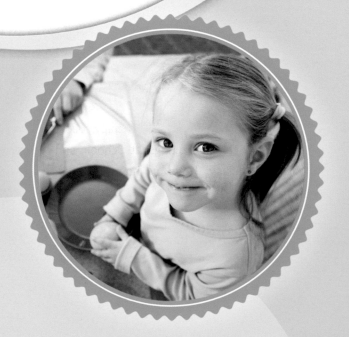

Where to Start?

One of the reasons I was eager to update the *Special Diets* books was because I wanted to discuss a healthier way of feeding a family. This goes for children not on restricted diets too, but with everything on your plate, that might seem like an impossible goal.

It goes without saying that the parents of children with autism are overwhelmed most of the time. There is always something that needs to be done — speech therapy, occupational therapy, meetings at school, and in-home therapy. There are homework sessions to supervise (for all the children in the family), and sports and other extra-curricular activities to attend (and for which you are also the chauffeur!). I know how hard this is, how exhausting and stressful it is, because I have been there and done that! Unlike many of the other authors of "special" cookbooks, I too

have both a son on the autism spectrum and one who is not. I have done it while working full-time outside the home, and while working on my own terms from a home office. Either way, it is stressful and draining.

So I can understand why it seems more reasonable to bring food in or take the family out. I can understand the desire to pop open a can or reheat a frozen meal in the microwave. But (you knew there would be a *but*) I believe that you can feed your family better quality meals while expending no more energy than it takes to load everyone into the car, drive to a restaurant, and hope to heaven that no one melts down or has a crisis!

Why do I believe this? Because it is true once you learn my special mantra: *simplify*. There it is … say it softly to yourself. Repeat it in a rhythm until you feel your muscles relaxing. That is it! The secret to healthy, home-cooked meals. How can you do this? Trust me, it is easier than you think. Simplify!

⊚ **Cook beef, poultry, and fish without fancy breading or stuffing.** Season meat with salt, pepper, the herbs your family likes, and perhaps a squeeze of lemon. Cook it on top of the stove, in the oven, or (better yet) on the grill. If your children do not want to eat chicken that has not been breaded and fried, hold your ground. It is unlikely they will starve. Once they are used to the new form that chicken comes in, they will find that it is good. Only then should you bother with the occasional (homemade) nugget. You will be teaching your family to eat protein that is not covered in starch, and you will be lowering grain intake and calories, too. If you can afford to buy organic, free-range chicken, you should do so. If you cannot, then buy poultry that has not been injected with anything. There should be only one ingredient — chicken. If you can afford to buy organic grass-fed beef, do so. If it is out of your budget, consider buying a cow or part of one. We order a portion of the cow in the spring, and when it arrives in early summer, we have enough meat to last the year. Since my family has shrunk, I am down to ⅙ of a cow. However,

for a bigger family, a whole cow or larger fraction will be necessary. The price of this beef is far less than I would pay for conventional beef in my store, and about one-half what I would pay for grass-fed. The only requirement is somewhere to put the meat — a basement or garage freezer is a must!

⊚ **Serve fresh fruit *every day*.** More children like fruit than vegetables, and there is excellent nutrition to be found in fruits if you vary them and do not use the same two or three fruits every day. Be sure that you are adding berries and other fruits naturally high in antioxidants. Add tropical fruits to mix things up, and be sure to eat your own fruit with gusto and obvious enjoyment. What could be simpler? There is nothing to cook — just slice it up and serve it. Serve one fruit or use a few to make a fruit salad. If your children refuse to eat fruit, blend it into smoothies and frozen pops for now, but keep offering whole or sliced fruit regularly. Pretend you will not share your wonderful peach, and someone just might beg for a bite. If you have a high speed blender, such as Vitamix, unsweetened frozen fruit can be turned into a sorbet or frozen yogurt (using coconut yogurt) in less than 10 minutes.

⊚ **Be sure that your children eat their veggies *every day*.** Children who do not like vegetables will often eat them if there is a tasty dip or zesty salsa available. Make sure that kid-sized vegetable sticks are readily available for snacking. If they do not like common vegetables, such as carrots, try something like jicama or turnip. Sometimes children prefer a vegetable with a little flavor to a bland celery stick. When you are trying to get your children to eat vegetables, consider buying baby veggies — they are generally less bitter and children like kid-sized foods. Drizzle them with olive oil and salt and roast at 375°F for about 20 minutes — this brings out the sweetness of the vegetables. Blanch fresh vegetables, or steam them quickly to preserve nutrients and vibrant color.

If they still refuse them, blend vegetables and add them to casseroles and soups, or make green smoothies (see chapter 4). If you must sneak vegetables in, be sure to reintroduce them in their more natural state regularly. Serve vegetables year-round! When spring and summer roll around, buy fresh local produce whenever possible. Your local farmer's market is a great place to buy your vegetables, but do not assume that cold weather means the end to good vegetables. Most people think that frozen vegetables are second-rate, but they are often better tasting and more nutritious than the fresh produce at your store. How can this be? Well, vegetables lose nutrients starting the moment they are picked. There is no way to know when the vegetables in the grocery store were picked, how long they sat in a truck, and how long they took to get to you. Frozen vegetables, on the other hand, are picked and frozen quickly before they lose many vitamins and minerals.

⑤ **Keep starches to a minimum.** Even if your child is not on a carbohydrate restricted diet, it is a good goal to reduce the number of carbohydrates being eaten. Later, if you decide to try SCD, you will have an easier time making the switch. One of the easiest ways to reduce starches is to serve them only infrequently for breakfast. American breakfasts tend to be starch-heavy (e.g., cereal, toast, pancakes, waffles, muffins). However, what a child really needs to start the day is a serving of protein. As discussed in chapter 5, leftover dinner food makes a great breakfast and solves this problem with no fuss and little cooking. Since most of the starchy foods that your child can eat will require baking from scratch or a mix (or at the very least a trip to a natural foods store), limiting starches will help you achieve the goal to *simplify*.

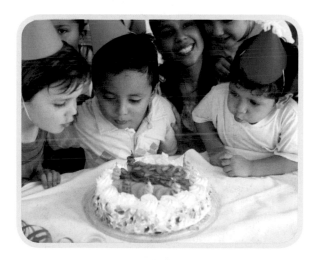

⑤ **Remember that cookies, cakes, and other sweets are for holidays, birthdays, and special occasions.** Sticking to this will help your children in many ways. They will learn to satisfy their sweet cravings with fruit instead of cookies. They will reduce their reliance on refined sugars and empty calories. When sweets are rarely eaten, previously loved treats often become "too sweet," and you may be able to lower the sugar even when you are making sweets. Limiting treats also helps you simplify since you will not be baking nearly as often, and you will not be buying expensive cookie and cake substitutes.

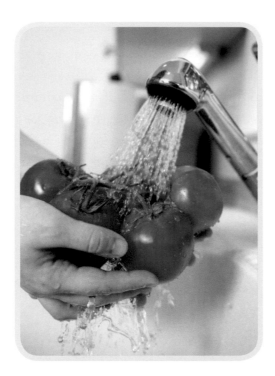

Other Tips

⑤ Do not store fruit and vegetables together. Ripening fruit emits ethylene gas, which can affect the flavor of vegetables.

⑤ Although convenient, tomatoes are so acidic that they leach harmful chemicals (such as BPA) from the aluminum can. Some brands are sold in glass jars or vacuum packs (e.g., Pomi). A few brands use enamel-lined cans, which are safe. These include Eden Organic and Trader Joe's. Muir Glen, a subsidiary of General Mills, is in the process of switching to BPA-free cans, and should be safe to use in the near future. Call the company to find out if they have completed the switch before buying this brand.

⑤ Buying organic — is it important or a waste of money? That depends … some conventional foods are fine, and you do not need to spend extra on organic versions. Others, however, are worth the extra expense. The Environmental Working Group has developed a Shopper's Guide to Pesticides that lists the "Dirty Dozen" and the "Clean 15." Among the worst (dirtiest) foods are peaches, berries, nectarines, cherries, apples, and some greens. The clean list includes onions, avocado, pineapple, and melons. Download the free guide from www.foodnews.org (they even have an "app" for your iPhone). Whenever you bring home fruit or vegetables (conventional or organic), be sure to wash them carefully with a specially developed fruit wash. These food soaps are available at most natural food stores.

Ingredients to Avoid

Everyone tells you to avoid processed foods. I often say that if it takes more than 5 seconds to read the ingredient list, put it back. Seriously though, when you read those lists, it is fairly shocking. Since I know you will be simplifying, and you will not be using processed foods, this should not be a problem. But if you do buy some prepared foods, try to avoid these ingredients:

⑤ Artificial Colors: Previously made from coal tar, these are now mostly petroleum-based products. Do we really want to feed them to our families? If you need to color a food, see "Spritz Cookies" recipe on page 258.

⑤ Artificial Flavors: These are lab-created flavors designed to mimic real food flavor and trick our brains. It is much better to use real food with real flavors.

⑤ Artificial Sweeteners: These are discussed at some length in chapter 13. Suffice it to say that the chemically derived non-caloric sweeteners found in diet foods and soda have been linked to cancer, dizziness, seizures, and headaches.

⑤ Artificial Preservatives: These include (but are not limited to) butylated hydroxytoluene (BHT), butylated hydroxyanisole (BHA), tert-butylhydroquinone (TBHQ), and all benzoate chemicals designed to preserve fats and keep food from becoming rancid. They have been linked to hyperactivity, asthma, and skin conditions, and may affect estrogen levels.

⑤ High Fructose Corn Syrup: This ubiquitous "food" is a cheap alternative to table sugar. It is used to sweeten foods, but also contributes to browning and sustains freshness in baked foods. It may predispose the body to turn fructose into fat, and increases the risk for type-II diabetes.

⑤ Monosodium Glutamate (MSG): This flavor enhancer is used in many restaurants, and is also commonly added to processed foods. The culprit behind "Chinese Restaurant Syndrome," MSG causes headaches, dizziness, and wheezing in susceptible individuals. It may also lead to weakness, breathing difficulties, and burning sensations.

⑤ Partially Hydrogenated Fats: These man-made fats are used in thousands of processed foods because they are cheap and very stable. They contain high levels of trans fats that raise low-density lipoprotein (bad cholesterol [LDL]) and lower high-density lipoprotein (good cholesterol [HDL]).

How to Go GFCF

Because it is generally easier to eliminate all dairy products from the diet than to remove all traces of gluten, many people decide to eliminate dairy first, then gluten later. There are many milk substitutes, but be sure that you choose one that is also gluten-free. Even if you attempt to make this a gradual change, it makes no sense to have your child adjust to a substitute that will not be used later.

Although soy "milks" are easy to find, this is not a good choice for a milk substitute. Many children are also allergic or sensitive to soy, and those who are sensitive to casein usually react to soy as well. There are now other excellent choices such as unsweetened rice, almond, or coconut milk. Health food stores generally carry all three, either in vacuum-sealed packs or in the refrigerator section. DariFree™ is potato-based, and is a good choice if you are not avoiding all starch.

Many of these beverages come in powdered or liquid form — although the liquid is more convenient for drinking, you will want to have powder on hand, too. Many of the GF bread recipes (e.g., nearly all those in Bette Hagman's books) call for powdered milk. The

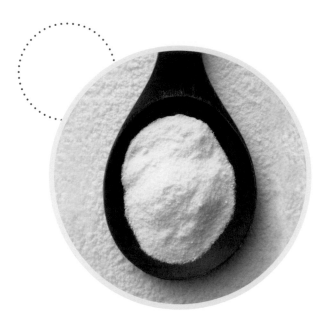

powdered form is also easy to use in recipes that call for liquid milk. For every cup of milk substitute in the recipe, add 8 ounces water to the wet ingredients, and 2–3 tablespoons dry powdered substitute to the dry ingredients.

As you might expect, all the milk substitutes cost more than cow's milk, and the powdered form is generally less expensive than the liquid. Many brands can be purchased by the case or in large tubs — buying in bulk almost always saves money.

Turtle Mountain has recently introduced a line of yogurts made from coconut milk. Because it is cultured, it contains the same types of probiotics that you would find in dairy yogurt. The plain variety contains 30% of the RDA for calcium. This wonderful coconut yogurt is sold under the label "So Delicious" and is available at natural food stores and many groceries. This yogurt is great for snacking or adding to a lunch box, but it also makes great dips, dressings, and frozen desserts.

When a recipe calls for butter or shortening, there are many options available. My favorite products are from Earth Balance. They make a line of GFCF spreads that contain no trans-fats or partially hydrogenated oils. Read the ingredients — some products contain soy. They have spreads that come in tubs, and sticks for cooking and baking.

Another choice is coconut oil, or coconut butter, as it is sometimes called. While we are accustomed to thinking of any saturated fat as unhealthy, unprocessed coconut oil is unlikely to raise cholesterol levels. Coconut oil is a medium chain fatty acid; because it is naturally saturated, it does not have to be hydrogenated to solidify at room temperature. It is the process of hydrogenation that creates trans fats. Trans fats raise the bad cholesterol (LDL) and lower the good cholesterol (HDL) levels. Long chain fatty acids, which are stored as fat in the body, are associated with cholesterol problems. Further, approximately one-half the fatty acid of coconut oil is lauric acid. A component of human milk, lauric acid has antibacterial, antiviral and antifungal properties. It is also a source of Medium Chain Triglycerides (MCTs), which allow the body to metabolize fat efficiently and convert it to energy rather than storing it as fat. For cooking or baking, replace butter or margarine with three-quarters the amount of coconut oil.

I am often asked if goat's milk, yogurt, or cheeses are acceptable for this diet. According to Dr. Karl Reichelt (Reichelt, et al., 1981; Knivsberg, et al., 1990; Knivsberg, et al., 1994), the casein in goat (and sheep) milk is very similar to that of cow's milk and should be avoided. My son is very sensitive to gluten, but does not seem to react to casein. I try to keep milk products out of his diet, because of the similarity between the casein and gluten molecules, but occasional use of goat's cheese and yogurt has not caused a perceptible reaction. According to Reichelt, if your child showed developmental problems from a very early age (infancy), you should avoid *all* dairy products.

If foods, like countries, were afforded "most favored" status, cheese would certainly qualify. I can honestly say I have never met a child who did not like cheese. Foods with cheese, such as pizza and macaroni and cheese, have been standards of childhood for generations. Until recently, there really was no decent cheese substitute, but that has changed! Daiya makes a terrific GFCF cheese substitute. Available in cheddar and mozzarella style shreds, this "cheese" melts, stretches, and even tastes like cheese.

On to Gluten...

Removing gluten from the diet tends to be a bit trickier (and more labor intensive) than removing casein. Many of our children are addicted to wheat-based snacks: breads, muffins, pretzels, crackers, and noodles. The goal for most parents should be to greatly reduce reliance on these starchy foods, and increase proteins, fresh fruits, and vegetables. However, this is probably a gradual process. In the meantime, you can find substitutes for some of your child's favorite wheat snacks.

GFCF breads are available at all health food stores and many groceries. The Food for Life rice-almond, rice-pecan, and rice breads are quite good. They are generally available in the freezer case of health food stores. Ener-G sells several types of GFCF and yeast-free breads. They are vacuum packed and can be found on the shelf or in the freezer of most natural food stores, and are also available through mail order. Although they make acceptable toast and bread crumbs, they are not, in my opinion, very tasty. If yeast is being avoided, these breads are often the only available option.

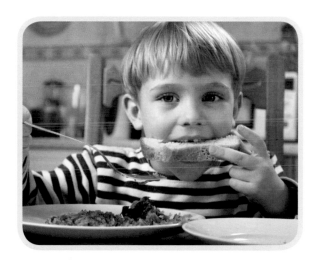

If yeast must be avoided but your child refuses to eat the commercially available loaves, try making sandwiches using quick breads. Be sure to cut back on the amount of sugar so that they are more bread-like than cake-like. You can also use GF waffles for sandwiches. For those avoiding all grains, there are several good recipes on the SCD support site, Pecanbread.com.

There are many GF **crackers** on the market; visit a store with a good selection of GF foods and read the labels carefully. There are many excellent mixes for **breads** and other baked foods available. See chapter 5 for brands and online sources. There are many excellent GF **pastas** available through mail order or in natural food stores. Pastas made from quinoa and rice, in various shapes and sizes, can be found easily. These will serve as excellent substitutes for wheat noodles in all your recipes. Of course, pasta is a starchy food, so use it in moderation.

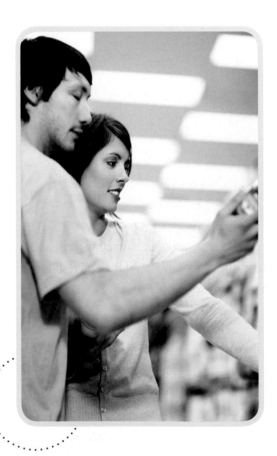

Shop the Ethnic Aisle

America is often called a "melting pot," and this cultural diversity is beneficial to many of us searching for recipes that will fit our child's special dietary needs. An easy way to vary the diet is by borrowing from other ethnic cultures, especially those that are rice-based. Go to the library and check out cookbooks on Chinese, Japanese, Thai, Korean, and Indian cuisine. You will find that many of the recipes will not require any modifications.

Even familiar foods, such as rice, are prepared differently in distant parts of the world. Short-grain rice (known as Arborio rice) is easy to find — Italians use it to cook risotto. It has a wonderful creamy texture that most children, even finicky ones, like. It can be varied in hundreds of ways; whole cookbooks have been dedicated to its preparation.

In many Mexican dishes, rice and beans are combined in delicious recipes that contain high-quality protein and no forbidden foods. Asian, Indian, and Hispanic grocery stores are wonderful sources of unusual or hard-to-find ingredients. In addition to carrying white rice flour and sweet rice flour, Asian markets also carry many types of rice noodles and rice wrappers. These wrappers are brittle, but when dipped in water for a few moments, they become soft and pliable. They can then be filled with vegetables, meat, or a combination of both, and made into little egg rolls or wontons. Indian stores often sell rice flakes (poha), which can be used much like oatmeal. Because poha is crunchier than rolled oats, you may prefer to add it to a recipe's wet ingredients for a few minutes to soften.

Hispanic markets also have ingredients that can be used to vary and enliven the diet. Both **plantain and coconut flours** make wonderful additions to breads, pancakes, and waffles. Many grocery stores also carry other items used in Spanish and Puerto Rican cuisine, especially if the neighborhood is ethnically mixed. If you can find such a store, look carefully at items that are unfamiliar to you. In addition to many rice, lentil, and bean products, you can also find unusual vegetables. The store I shop at carries fresh and frozen taro, malanga, and cassava — all of which can be cooked and eaten like potatoes. Because these tubers (root vegetables) are fairly bland, they can serve as the base of many interesting dishes. They are also suitable for a white diet if you are trying to eliminate all (or nearly all) pigments.

Malanga is often considered to be the most hypoallergenic food in the world because its starch grains are the smallest and most easily digested of all complex carbohydrates. Even children with extreme sensitivities should tolerate it. Malanga is closely related to the **taro** root, which is used to make poi in many Polynesian cultures. **Cassava** (also known as manioc) is a large brown root that is white and fleshy on the inside. Tapioca, which most people are familiar with, is derived from this root. **Cassava must be cooked before eating** — it is toxic when raw. Flours made from these and other unusual foods can be obtained via mail order. (See Appendix I.)

Baking from Scratch — Without Gluten

Though I am encouraging less reliance on baked foods, there are times when you will want to make muffins or cookies. To do so successfully requires that you understand the function gluten serves in baked goods.

Gluten is an elastic protein. When you are making bread, the process of kneading the dough develops the gluten, creating stretchy strands. The gases given off by the metabolism of the yeast get trapped in the spaces created by this "web" of dough, and push the dough up and out. (In other words, the dough rises.)

In non-yeast breads and cookies, the dough is not kneaded; in fact, overmixing muffins or quick-bread batter will begin to develop the gluten, which is undesirable. Developing the gluten in quick breads or muffins will result in holes and tunnels, and will make beautiful pancakes that are tough rather than tender. But even in these foods, the stretchiness of the gluten provides the necessary structure to prevent a cookie from disintegrating into crumbs the instant you pick it up.

Since the GF flours and flour combinations do not contain gluten, something else must serve the same function if the end result is to be acceptable. This is possible with the addition of **xanthan gum, methylcellulose, or guar gum**. These ingredients can be hard to find — most health food stores carry at least one of them (typically xanthan gum). If you cannot find any of these at your local health food store, most of the mail-order companies carry one or more of them. Guar gum has a laxative effect for some people, so xanthan gum is generally preferable. It is expensive, but because it is used sparingly, a little goes a long way. When converting a recipe to GF flour, add 1 to 1½ teaspoons xanthan gum for each cup of flour. Many GF bakers also add 1–3 teaspoons egg replacement powder, powdered pectin, or unflavored gelatin to their breads.

These ingredients improve the texture of breads. The texture of a baked product, often called the "mouth feel," is important. Although you may not consciously notice the crumb structure and "mouth feel" when you eat a slice of bread or a piece of cake, these are factors that contribute to whether or not you enjoy the food. If you think back to some wonderful food you ate in the past, most likely you will recall the sensation of having it in your mouth — perhaps you remember that it was "silky" or "velvety." If everyone notices these factors on some level, imagine how important such textural characteristics are for children (or adults) who have tactile defensiveness or other sensory disturbances.

To achieve both pleasant tastes and textures in your quick breads, cookies, cakes, yeast breads, and muffins, you will need to keep a variety of flours on hand. If you have never tried living without gluten, many of the flours will be unfamiliar to you. Some are native to the United States but used mainly for livestock or as fillers; others are borrowed from different cultures. For the most part, you will want to combine more than one type of flour when you bake without gluten.

GF Flours

If you have a favorite recipe that is usually made with wheat flour, you will probably be able to modify it for the GFCF diet. You will need to use one (or a combination) of the GF flours that follow, and you must add 1 teaspoon xanthan gum (or one of the other gluten substitutes) for each cup of flour. Generally, you will also want to add structure by increasing the number of eggs in the recipe — if you want to avoid too much fat use only the egg whites for the additional egg(s), or use an egg replacer powder.

Often an increase in leavening is required when a recipe is modified for GF flours. An extra ½ teaspoon baking powder or baking soda may be sufficient, but to be sure, you will need to experiment a bit. Another way to improve the results of baked goods using these flours is to make smaller loaves or cakes. You can divide a quick-bread batter between two mini-loaf pans, or you could make rolls instead of a loaf. Larger baked products certainly can be made, but the smaller ones are often more like the real thing in texture.

Because different flours absorb different amounts of liquid, you may have to use more or less liquid in a recipe, depending on your choice of flour. The consistency of your dough or batter is what counts; try to achieve the consistency described in a recipe by adjusting the liquid. In general, use only part of the liquid called for, adding the full amount if needed. If the mixture is still too dry or too heavy, add more than the recipe called for, a few tablespoons at a time.

It is helpful to make notes as you experiment so you will not forget which modification produced the best outcome. You may need to make more than one modification, and it may take a few trials. However, in most cases, you can duplicate your family's favorites fairly reliably.

GF Flour Blend

In general, you cannot go wrong with Bette Hagman's GF Flour Blend. This mix consists of:

2 parts white rice flour

⅔ part potato starch flour

⅓ part tapioca starch flour

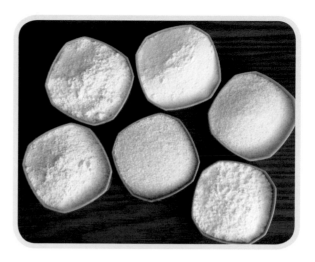

With 1 teaspoon xanthan gum added per cup of flour mix, GF flours can be used as a direct substitute for white flour in nearly any recipe. You should keep some of this mixture on hand at all times; it is easy to mix up a large canister yourself. If you prefer, Ener-G sells it in 1- and 5-pound packages. It is available at many health food stores or through mail order. There are also other companies that make GF flour blends that you might like. I often use the 365 brand available at Whole Foods, or Bob's Red Mill brand. See chapter 5 for suggestions.

Quinoa Flour

Quinoa is a GF flour that adds good body and flavor to baked goods; if used alone it tastes rather odd, so use it for no more than one-half the flour in a given recipe. (Some celiac groups contend that quinoa is not gluten-free, but most agree that it is a safe food.)

Rice Flours

Brown and white rice flours are the basis of most GF baking. Brown rice flour contains more nutrients since it is less refined, and it is sometimes easier to find since many health food stores have a "no refined products" policy. For making cakes, breads, and cookies, however, you need white rice flour. Arrowhead Mills makes one; since almost all health food stores (and many supermarkets) carry this brand, you should be able to get the store manager to order the white rice variety. Be warned, however, that this brand is not nearly as soft as some others (such as Ener-G), and some children may not tolerate the somewhat grainy feel of foods made with this flour. Many stores carry bags of white rice flour made by Goya; this is a very soft, fine flour that will work well in GF baking. Asian markets are also good sources for soft white rice flour. **Sweet rice flour** makes an excellent thickener for gravies or cream sauces. Sometimes called "glutinous" flour, it does not contain any gluten.

Jowar Flour

Jowar flour is another excellent GF alternative. This flour is made from sorghum; many people say that, with xanthan gum added, it is interchangeable with wheat flour in most recipes. It is darker and heartier than rice flours — I would suggest using it in recipes that call for whole wheat flour. In general, I would recommend using jowar for only part of the flour in a given recipe; when used alone the end product tends to be quite heavy. American farmers grow sorghum, and there are a few American companies that sell it. It is usually available at Indo-Pak groceries, and is generally cheaper there.

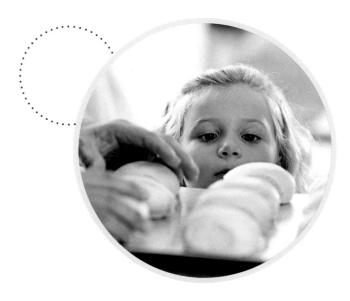

Potato Starch Flour

Potato starch flour is available in health food stores and in the kosher section of most supermarkets. Do not confuse potato **starch** flour with potato flour. The latter has a heavy flavor, and the two cannot be used interchangeably in recipes. **Tapioca starch flour** is also widely available, and has a texture similar to **corn starch**. In fact, if your child is sensitive to corn, tapioca starch flour makes a good substitute. **Arrowroot** is a starch with similar properties, and I have yet to hear of a child who cannot tolerate it. This starch makes an excellent addition to waffle and pancake recipes — giving the finished product an excellent texture, soft inside yet crispy on the outside. Another alternative starch is **kuzu root starch**, made from the wild kuzu plant; it is rich in minerals, and some people prefer it to arrowroot and other starches.

Bean Flours

Bean flours, such as pea, lentil, or chickpea, combine well with rice flour, and are excellent ingredients for breading. Foods made with white rice flour contain very little protein, but adding bean flour will significantly increase the protein content of your baked goods. They can also be added to meat for binding when making burgers or meatballs. Indian cuisine uses chickpea flour (besan) to make a batter for dipping and frying vegetables (pakoras). Lentil flour is the main ingredient for small Indian breads called pappadam; these are crunchy and delicious. Pappadam mixes can be found at Indo-Pak groceries. They are also available pre-formed; to prepare them you need only fry in oil for a few minutes just before serving (they can also be baked).

Poi Flour

Poi flour (taro) is extremely digestible and is excellent if there are multiple allergies or gastrointestinal problems. It is a good source of Vitamin B-1 and calcium. It can be made into hot cereal or used as a thickener for soups or puddings.

Montina

Montina is a relative newcomer to the GF flour world. Made of Indian ricegrass, this GF grain is unrelated to rice. Amazing Grains makes a bread flour and an all-purpose flour blend; it can be ordered online through Amazon.com. For more information, visit www.amazing-grains.com.

The Importance of Eggs

Eggs serve many functions in baking, but unfortunately, many children simply cannot tolerate them. While many egg substitutes exist, you must first determine the function of the egg in a particular recipe before you can decide which one is appropriate. For most recipes, Ener-G egg substitute will work well. This and similar products are made of potato starch, tapioca flour, and baking powder, and are well tolerated by most people. If egg serves as a leavening agent, 1 teaspoon baking powder for each egg in the recipe should work. In cakes, 1 teaspoon vinegar can be used for each egg — this also serves as a leavening agent.

If egg is being used as a binder in muffins or quick breads, you can boil 1 tablespoon flax seed or flax seed powder in a cup of water for 15 minutes, and add this as needed to your batter. Flax seeds can also be ground and added directly to baked goods — they add fiber and are an excellent source of essential fatty acids. Another way to replace eggs is to soften 1 teaspoon gelatin in 3 tablespoons boiling water. Stir until the gelatin is completely dissolved and freeze until it has thickened a bit. Beat until frothy; this equals one egg.

Of course, nothing gives baked goods the structure and moistness of real egg — if you know the culprit to avoid is the egg yolk, egg whites are fine. For every egg needed, use two whites. If the egg white must be avoided, I would recommend using extra yolks only when real egg is preferable (i.e., in cakes). The yolk is high in fat and cholesterol, so a substitution rather than doubling up on yolks would be advisable. If an egg allergy exists, be aware that an egg by any other name is still an egg! When you read labels, watch out for ingredients such as albumin, conalbumin, livetin, mucoid, ovomucoid, ovalbumin, and vitellin — these product ingredients are all derived from egg.

Using the Senses in GFCF Baking

Eating involves most of our senses, with input coming to many different sensory channels at the same time. The way in which our brain interprets these sensory experiences greatly influences how we feel about particular foods. To enjoy (or even try) a food, it must first be *visually* appealing to us. If we do not like the *smell* of a food, it is unlikely we will be willing to eat it. It has to *feel* right too; I have never liked pears as much as other fruits, because they are too grainy and I dislike the sensation against my teeth and tongue. If a child finds a food too hard or too chewy, it may seem like too much trouble to eat. And of course, if we are to enjoy a food, it does have to *taste* good, too.

It should not be surprising that some of these senses also give us important information as we are baking. If you are aware of your senses, you will have more baking success whether you are using wheat or GF flours. For example, here is an old baker's trick you

should be aware of: Let yourself be led by your nose! Always open the oven to check for doneness when you *first* begin to smell your bread, cake, cookies, or muffins. Good smells begin to emerge from your oven when the food is *almost* baked through; if you can smell it, the food should be closely monitored from that point on. Most of us do not notice those first aromas; by the time we smell the

food, it is often a bit overbaked — too dark or too dry.

Believe it or not, if you really pay attention to your sense of smell while you are baking, you can train yourself to start noticing those first aromas. After a while this comes naturally, and you will not need to concentrate on it. At first you may only notice the smell when the food is actually done (or overdone). Soon, however, you will start noticing those aromas sooner when foods are not quite baked through. If the food looks done on the outside, but is still raw inside, cover the pan with foil sprayed with cooking spray and continue to test every 5 minutes.

Another sensory trick that works well with cakes, quick breads, and muffins involves your *hearing*. Listen to your food! I know that sounds strange, but if a cake looks quite done and the toothpick test is equivocal (perhaps it tests very moist but not actually wet), hold the pan up to your ear and listen. A cake or quick bread that is still uncooked will have a steady, continuous crackling sound that is rather loud when held close to the ear. A cake that is moist, but not wet inside, will emit a much softer crackle. (A silent cake is probably going to be very dry.) If listening to cakes sounds crazy, try this: The next time you bake a cake, take it out of the oven when you are sure it needs another 15–20 minutes of baking. Hold the cake up to your ear and listen for a few moments, then return it to the oven and bake until it tests done. When you remove the finished cake from the oven, listen to it again. From that point on, you will be able to recognize the difference quite easily.

If you want to prepare freshly baked bread, but just cannot bring yourself to start from scratch, try some of the excellent mixes available from the mail-order companies listed in chapter 5. Most of these mixes are easy to make, and the results are delicious. They are a good compromise between store-bought and homemade. Even if you like to bake from scratch, a few mixes are wonderful to have on hand for those days when you are simply too busy. Many people on GF diets use only the mixes; they do not like baking, and this is a good solution for them.

Breakfast and Breads

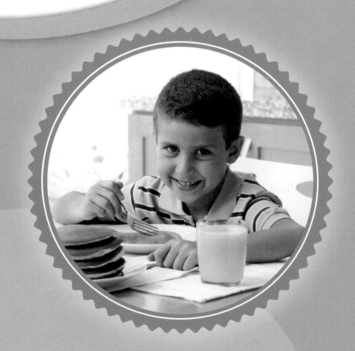

For many people just beginning to cook for special diets, breakfast seems to be the easiest meal to manage. Most children like the usual breakfast foods — muffins, pancakes, waffles, and toast (although eggs are often not a favorite). Unfortunately, the versions of these foods that our children have grown up on are generally wheat- and dairy-based, and loaded with sugar. In addition, they are often very low in protein, which children need to start their day and succeed in school.

While many families have an occasional "breakfast for dinner," few reverse that trend and eat dinner for breakfast. This would never have occurred me to when I was a child (one who ate cereal and milk every day of the year). My children, on the other hand, have always loved dinner leftovers for breakfast. It may seem strange at first to give your children left-over grilled chicken for breakfast, but really, is it so odd? In most cultures breakfast foods are no different from food served at other meals. In big hotels in Asia, "western breakfasts" are available for tourists, but that is not what you would find at a family's breakfast table. When

I finally figured this out, I began to make extra dinner and set it aside for breakfast, especially if I was serving something that was a particular favorite.

I would love to see people serve leftover beef or chicken with some fruit for breakfast, rather than loading up on heavily sweetened carbohydrates. Some children just will not will not will not eat any other kind of breakfast though, and if you are creative (and learn to hide nutrients), traditional breakfast foods can be reasonably healthy.

The following recipes for quick breads, muffins, pancakes, biscuits, and rolls should help get you started. Be sure to review chapter 3 for general tips on baking with GFCF ingredients.

When baking muffins, fill the muffin cups of your pan as directed. Any empty cups should be filled with ¼–½ cup water. This

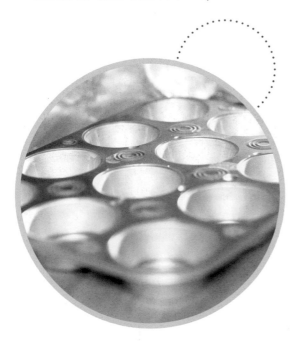

helps the muffins stay moist and prevents the pan from warping.

Muffin top pans can be found wherever muffin tins are sold, and make only the rounded top. They have the added advantage of making small muffins, which look a little bit like fat cookies. If you use these pans, you will need to decrease baking time a little since the volume of batter is smaller.

I have not included any yeast-bread recipes since so many people avoid yeast. For a huge assortment of wonderful GF yeast breads, I recommend *The Gluten-Free Gourmet* book series by the late Bette Hagman, which is published by Holt.

If a recipe calls for GF flour mix, it means that I make it with the Hagman GF flour mix. You can mix this up yourself, or you can buy it already mixed. There are other excellent GF flour mixes available such as Bob's Red Mill brand and the Whole Foods GF flour. The recipes will also work with these commercially prepared flour blends. There are also mixtures that include beans and some flours that work well as a one-to-one substitute for wheat (e.g., sorghum). These recipes will work with pretty much any flour mixture, but remember that different kinds of flours absorb different volumes of liquid. Try to get the consistency as described in the recipe, which may mean using a little more or less water or milk substitute. It is often advisable to use a little less than the full amount of liquid, adding more as needed, to achieve the proper consistency of the batter or dough.

Note that when a recipe calls for milk substitute, it is referring to liquid; when powdered milk substitute is required, the recipe will specify. For recipes calling for maple syrup, be sure to use pure syrup, not the corn syrup and flavoring concoctions sold under the big brand names. Or make mock syrup by adding a few drops of a strong maple flavoring to 100% pure vegetable glycerin. (This can be used to lightly sweeten foods for a yeast-free diet.)

When I first began to bake gluten-free, I only used alcohol-free flavorings, fearing that the alcohol in a typical extract might contain some gluten. We now know that gluten is not present in detectable amounts in vanilla and other extracts, and I am comfortable using a good quality vanilla. Do not, however, use imitation vanilla or any food that contains vanillin.

Finally, it is worth noting that there are now many excellent mixes available in health food stores and online. Always read the ingredient list carefully, but the choices are wide and many are excellent. For the stressed and time-challenged parent, these can be a lifesaver. I also recommend making muffins, waffles, and pancakes in large amounts. They freeze well, and you can pull them out the night before and they will be ready to go in the morning. There are now prepared breakfast foods that were not widely available when *Special Diets* was first published, and some are quite good. Van's frozen waffles are excellent and can be found in most grocery stores. (Take care since not all of their products are gluten-free; their packages are well marked.)

Pancakes and Waffles

I cannot tell a lie — my family's favorite pancakes come from a mix! We all love the pancake and waffle mix made by the Canadian company, Kinnikinnick Foods. The mix contains a small amount of corn, which my son tolerates, but it does mean that many families would not be able to use it. There are other mixes available that might work for your family, too. Always read the ingredients and check with the company if you are in doubt. Here are some excellent recipes for pancakes, many of which were made popular following the first publication of *Special Diets*. Remember that nearly all will work for waffles, though you may need to decrease the liquid a little. ★

Karyn's Pancakes

ANDI Co-founder Karyn Seroussi created these pancakes, and points out that they make excellent crepes. To make crepes, decrease the flour to 1 cup.

1 Blend all ingredients except baking powder in a bowl. Add baking powder and stir just a few seconds to incorporate it into the batter.
2 Spoon on to a hot, oiled griddle and cook until bubbles form. Flip and cook on second side until done.
3 Serve with syrup or fruit.

Servings will vary.

1½ cups GF flour
   (buckwheat is excellent)
¾ cup powdered milk
   substitute (DariFree™ is
   recommended)
½ cup arrowroot powder
¼ cup sugar
2 eggs
1 tablespoon oil
¼ teaspoon salt
1 teaspoon GF baking powder

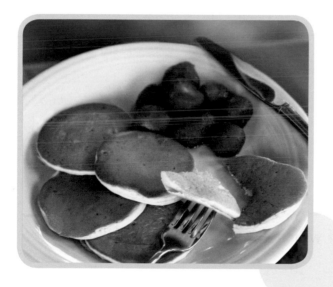

Don Baker's Pancakes

Dry Mixture

3 cups GF flour mix

3 tablespoons sugar

1 tablespoon GF baking
    powder

2 teaspoons xanthan gum

½ teaspoon salt

Wet Mixture

3 eggs

1¼ cups (or more) milk
    substitute

3 tablespoons oil
    (or melted CF margarine)

¼ teaspoon vanilla extract

This recipe is an old favorite that was first published in *Special Diets, Volume I*. These are tender and delicious, with just a little sweetness added. A few teaspoons of 100% pure vegetable glycerin would make this acceptable for a yeast-free diet. Extras freeze nicely.

1 Combine flour, sugar, baking powder, xanthan gum, and salt in a large bowl. Stir well.

2 Combine eggs, milk substitute, oil, and vanilla extract in a bowl and mix well.

3 Add to liquid mixture to dry mixture and stir until there are no bumps, but do not overmix. The batter should not be runny, but should plop from the spoon. If necessary, add more milk substitute, a little at a time, to reach this consistency.

4 Heat an oiled frying pan to high and drop batter in. Smaller pancakes are easier to turn, but if you prefer you can make large ones. Cook thoroughly until bubbles form and then flip to cook the second side until done.

5 Serve with fruit or maple syrup.

Servings will vary.

Banana (Nut) Pancakes

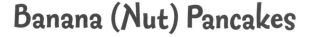

This is a recipe from the USA Rice Council. The nuts can be omitted if your family does not tolerate (or like) them. Because the only sweetener is honey, you could easily turn this into a recipe for a yeast-free diet by substituting 100% pure vegetable glycerin.

1 Combine flour, baking powder, salt, and xanthan gum in a medium bowl. Stir in water, oil, honey, egg yolks, bananas, and nuts.
2 Beat egg whites in another bowl, until stiff peaks form.
3 Fold egg whites into batter.
4 Bake pancakes on a hot, oiled griddle or frying pan. Cook on both sides until golden.

Servings will vary.

Hint: Separating the eggs, and beating the whites as directed, makes a lovely, light pancake. But if you are in a hurry, this step is not necessary. I often throw this batter together without beating the whites separately, and the result is still delicious.

1½ cups rice flour
2 teaspoons baking powder
1 teaspoon salt
½ teaspoon xanthan gum
1¼ cups water
3 tablespoons vegetable oil
2 tablespoons honey
2 eggs, yolks and whites separated
2 large bananas, mashed (or 1 [6-ounce] jar banana baby food)
½ cup chopped walnuts (optional)

✴ Easy Almond Flour Pancakes (SCD Pancakes)

1½ cups almond flour

5 eggs

1 tablespoon honey

1 teaspoon vanilla

½ teaspoon salt

¼ teaspoon GF baking soda

Ripe banana or any kind of berry (optional)

This recipe comes from Pam Ferro, RN. Pam is the head of the Gottschall Center in Mattapoisett, Massachusetts, and is an expert in grain-free diets.

1 Mix all ingredients in a bowl.

2 Cook on well-greased skillet on medium heat.

3 Drizzle with honey and serve.

Servings will vary.

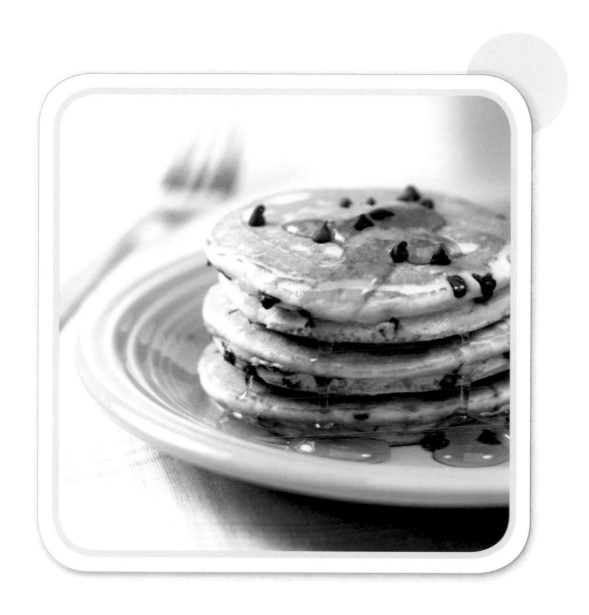

Muffins

Muffins are my favorite "vehicle" for hidden nutrients. First of all, most children love them and will eat them when nothing else appeals. If your children are little, you might try mini muffins; small foods that fit easily in little hands are often favorites. As for sneaking in nutrients — if eggs are tolerated—an extra egg white or some egg white powder adds protein.

Nuts also add protein and healthy fats, as well as crunch and flavor. If you take a few minutes to toast nuts first (see page 352), they taste even better. Many children think they do not like nuts, but it is usually the texture they dislike. Grinding them in a nut grinder (an inexpensive kitchen item) hides them beautifully. If you cannot find a nut grinder, a food processor will work, but be careful — process for too long and you will have nut butter.

You can also process or blend some carrots to add bulk, fiber, and vitamins without anyone realizing they are eating veggies. For a sweetener, a little molasses adds iron. Calcium powder and ground flax seeds also bump up the nutrition of muffins. (**Note:** Flax seed oil should not be used in baked goods since it loses healthful properties when heated.) ★

Karyn's Rice-Free Muffins

If your child is on a rotation diet, you need to be able to make some foods that contain no rice. This is another recipe from Karyn Seroussi, who created these when her son became sensitive to rice. If rice is not a problem, use brown rice instead of quinoa flour. This batter makes good pancakes, too.

1 Preheat oven to 350°F.

2 Combine flours, sugar, baking powder, xanthan gum, salt, and cinnamon in a bowl and set aside.

3 Beat together banana, eggs, milk substitute, and oil. Fold raisins into mixture.

4 Add liquid mixture to the dry ingredients and combine just until mixed.

5 Bake in an oiled muffin tin for approximately 15 minutes. Use a toothpick to check for doneness.

Makes 12 muffins

½ cup tapioca starch flour

½ cup quinoa flour

½ cup potato starch flour

⅓ cup sugar

2 teaspoons GF baking powder

I teaspoon xanthan gum

¼ teaspoon salt

½ teaspoon cinnamon (optional)

I banana, mashed

2 eggs

⅓ cup milk substitute or water

¼ cup oil

¼ cup raisins (optional)

Maple Rice-Bran Muffins

1¾ cups rice flour

¼ cup rice bran (available in health food stores)

1 tablespoon GF baking powder

½ teaspoon xanthan gum

½ teaspoon GF baking soda

¼ teaspoon salt

1 cup milk substitute

½ teaspoon lemon juice

2 eggs (or egg substitute or 4 egg whites)

3 tablespoons vegetable oil

⅓ cup pure maple syrup

1 cup apples, chopped (or pears)

1 cup raisins

1 teaspoon cinnamon

This is a recipe from the USA Rice Council. The original recipe calls for chopped apples, but pears can be substituted for those who must avoid apples. The recipe also calls for buttermilk — for a CF substitute, add ½ teaspoon lemon juice to 1 cup soy, rice, or potato milk. For yeast-free diets, alcohol-free maple flavoring could be added to 100% pure vegetable glycerin. Since children on yeast-free diets get so few treats, you might consider baking these muffins in colorful baking papers and calling them cupcakes!

1 Preheat oven to 425°F.

2 Combine flour, bran, baking powder, xanthan gum, baking soda, and salt in a large mixing bowl.

3 Whisk together milk substitute, juice, eggs, oil, and maple syrup in a medium bowl. Stir in apples, raisins, and cinnamon.

4 Make a well in the center of the dry mixture, pour liquid mixture into the well, and stir to combine.

5 Spoon batter into lightly greased muffin cups. Use back of wet spoon to smooth tops.

6 Bake for 18–20 minutes.

7 Cool on wire rack.

Makes 12 muffins

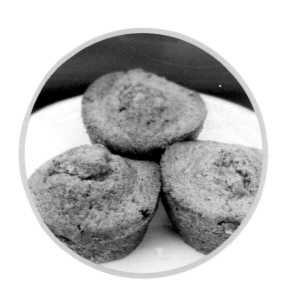

Blueberry Muffins

I love this recipe, which was given to me several years ago. I converted it to a muffin my son can eat, and it is almost as good as the original. I think you will like it too, even without real butter and whole wheat flour. The diced fruit adds moistness and extra flavor.

For the Muffins

1 Preheat oven to 350°F.
2 Grease bottoms only of muffin tins, or use lightly sprayed baking papers.
3 Beat eggs; stir in milk substitute, oil, and fruit in a bowl. Stir in cinnamon.
4 In a bowl, combine flour, brown sugar, xanthan gum, GF baking powder, and salt.
5 Stir dry mixture into liquid mixture until moistened (again, a few lumps are OK).
6 Spoon batter into muffin tins, filling about ⅔ full.

For the Topping

1 Combine ingredients in a small bowl, and sprinkle over the tops of muffins.
2 Bake for about 20 minutes, or until muffins test done.
3 Remove to wire rack at once to cool.

Makes 12 muffins

Muffins

1 egg, plus 1 egg white
1 cup milk substitute
    (soy or potato works best)
½ cup vegetable oil
1 tart pear, peeled and diced
1 cup fresh blueberries
½ teaspoon cinnamon
2 cups GF flour mix
⅓ cup brown sugar, packed
2 teaspoons xanthan gum
1 tablespoon, plus 1 teaspoon
    GF baking powder
1 teaspoon salt (optional)

Optional Topping

¼ cup brown sugar, packed
¼ cup pecans, chopped
½ teaspoon cinnamon

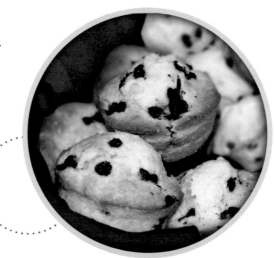

✳ *new* Grain-Free Blueberry Muffins

1½ cups coconut flour
1 cup nut flour
¼ cup honey
3 eggs, beaten
1 teaspoon vanilla extract
1 teaspoon pure lemon extract
½ teaspoon GF baking soda
½ teaspoon salt
1 cup blueberries

These muffins are dense and moist since they do not contain flour. They are a wonderful addition to a SCD diet, and are very tasty.

1 Preheat oven to 350°F.

2 Grease muffin tin or use liners. Mix all ingredients except blueberries until smooth in a bowl.

3 Fold blueberries into mixture.

4 Spoon batter into muffin tins, filling about ⅔ full.

5 Bake for about 20 minutes.

Makes 12 muffins

Variation: Add a sliced, ripe banana or finely diced apple or pear to the muffin batter.

Tropical Muffins

These muffins resulted from combining several recipes in my files. They are delicious for breakfast or as an afternoon snack.

1 Preheat oven to 400°F.

2 Grease or spray a muffin tin.

3 In a medium bowl, combine flour, sugar, baking powder, xanthan gum, and salt. Stir in chocolate chips and coconut.

4 In a smaller bowl, whisk together water, oil, eggs, powdered milk substitute, and orange flavor until light.

5 Add the liquid ingredients to the dry and stir together just until moistened and blended together. Do not overmix — a few lumps are OK.

6 Spoon batter into muffin tins, filling each ⅔ full.

7 Bake for about 15 minutes, rotating the tin back to front midway through baking. Remove when a toothpick inserted in the center comes out clean.

8 Cool on wire racks.

Makes 12 muffins

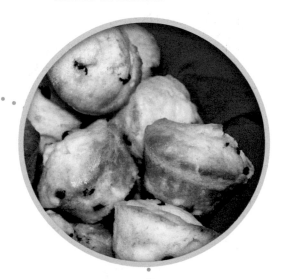

2 cups GF flour mix

⅓ cup sugar

3½ teaspoons GF baking powder

2 teaspoons xanthan gum

½ teaspoon salt

¾ cup GFCF mini chocolate chips* (Enjoy Life, Allergy Grocer, and Tropical Source are good brands)

½ cup shredded coconut (unsweetened, with no sulfites)

¾ cup water

⅓ cup vegetable oil

2 eggs

3 tablespoons powdered milk substitute

1½ teaspoons orange oil or flavoring (available from Williams-Sonoma)

*Chopped, dried fruit would be an excellent substitute for chocolate chips. Try pineapple or papaya to maintain the tropical mood.

Breads

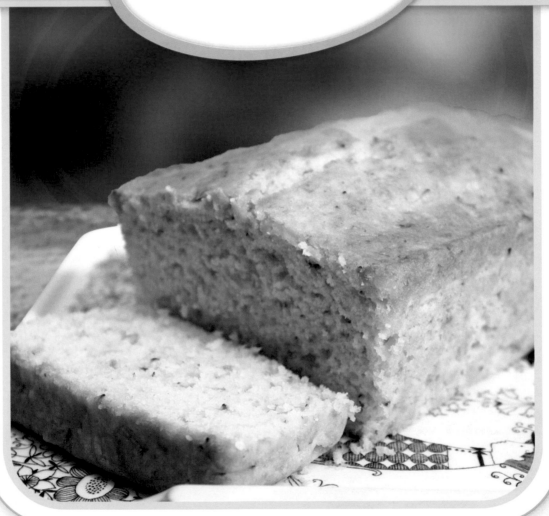

Food-Processor Zucchini Bread, recipe on page 76

Yeast-Free Sorghum Bread

Kelly Weaver is the source for this terrific bread. Sorghum flour (sometimes called jowar or juwar) is a wonderful addition to the GF kitchen. It works well in recipes developed for wheat flour and gives those on a rotation diet an additional choice. It is now fairly easy to find at the health food store. This recipe is special because it is hard to find a good yeast-free bread that slices and tastes like the real thing.

1 Preheat oven to 350°F.
2 Combine all ingredients in a bowl and mix well. Consistency will be a cake-like batter.
3 Grease and flour (with shortening and sorghum) a 9"x5"x3" bread pan.
4 Spoon batter into bread pan and bake for 30 minutes. Cover with foil and bake 25 minutes longer.
5 Remove loaf from pan and cool.

Makes 1 large loaf

2 cups sorghum flour
2 teaspoons GF baking powder
2 teaspoons dried egg whites
1½ teaspoons xanthan gum
½ teaspoon GF baking soda
½ teaspoon salt
2 eggs (or egg replacer and amount liquid suggested)
1 cup plus 1 tablespoon soda or sparkling water
3 tablespoons shortening* (Spectrum palm shortening, ghee, or GFCF margarine or oil)
2 tablespoons honey

Spectrum now makes a trans-fat–free solid shortening that can be used in place of Crisco or other hard shortenings. You could also use ghee, GFCF margarine, or oil in this recipe.

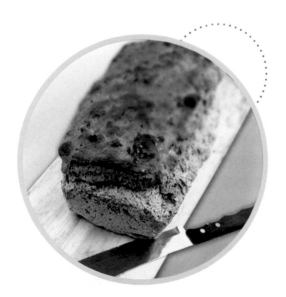

Food-Processor Zucchini Bread

I large zucchini

4 eggs

2 cups sugar

I cup oil
   (or ½ cup prune puree)

I teaspoon vanilla extract

3 cups GF flour mix

I tablespoon xanthan gum

I tablespoon cinnamon

I teaspoon salt

I teaspoon GF baking soda

I teaspoon GF baking powder

I cup walnuts, chopped
   (optional)

You need a food processor to make this delicious quick bread. If you do not have one, it will take some elbow grease to grate the zucchini, and a strong electric mixer to blend the batter. With a processor, this recipe is very simple. Like many quick breads, these are really more like cake than bread.

1 Preheat oven to 375°F.

2 Shred zucchini in a food processor.

3 Change to the steel blade and add eggs, sugar, oil, and vanilla. Mix well.

4 Mix together flour, xanthan gum, cinnamon, salt, baking soda, baking powder, and walnuts and add to the processor bowl. Process just until mixed.

5 Pour into two greased 9"x5"x3" loaf pans.

6 Bake for I hour or until breads test done.

Makes 2 large loaves

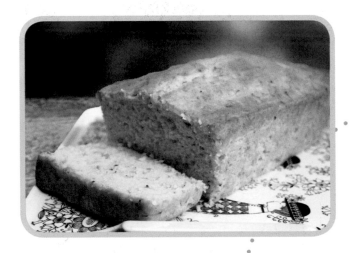

Coconut Quick Bread

This is delicious when served with Indian food, and can pass for dessert. It is an unusual bread, and one that you should try out on your family. Tip: toasted coconut improves the flavor of many quick breads — be sure to toast extra.

I cup grated coconut
   (with no sulfites)
2 cups GF flour mix
¾ cup sugar
I tablespoon baking powder
2 teaspoons xanthan gum
I cup milk substitute
   (soy works well)
2 eggs, beaten
¼ cup oil
I teaspoon vanilla extract

1 Preheat oven to 350°F.

2 Spread the coconut on a cookie sheet and toast until lightly browned. Watch carefully as coconut burns quickly. It should be light brown — stir once. This will take only 3–5 minutes.

3 Combine coconut with flour, sugar, baking powder, and xanthan gum in a bowl and mix well.

4 In a separate bowl, mix milk substitute, eggs, oil, and vanilla.

5 Add liquid mixture to dry mixture and blend well.

6 Pour into an oiled 9"x5"x3" loaf pan.

7 Bake for 50–60 minutes, until a toothpick inserted comes out clean and the bread is golden brown.

8 Cool completely and then store airtight.

Makes I large loaf

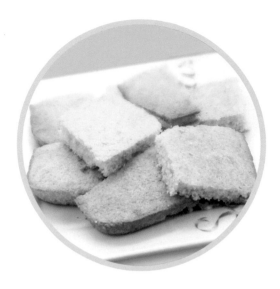

Sweet Corn Bread

This corn bread is similar to the version served at Boston Market restaurants. It can be used for tamale pie, but more often I use this batter for regular corn bread or for muffins.

1 Preheat oven to 400°F.

2 Blend together sugar and oil, then mix in eggs in a bowl.

3 In a separate bowl, mix flour, cornmeal, baking powder, xanthan gum, and salt well.

4 Blend dry ingredients into the egg mixture, alternating with milk substitute.

5 Bake in a 8"x8" greased square pan for 30 minutes, or until bread tests done. For muffins, check after 15 minutes.

Servings will vary.

¾ cup sugar

½ cup oil

2 eggs, lightly beaten

1½ cups GF flour blend (Hagman mix or soft rice flour)

1½ cups yellow cornmeal

1 tablespoon GF baking powder

1 teaspoon xanthan gum

⅛ teaspoon salt

1 cup milk substitute

Variation: if your family cannot eat corn, you can use a coarsely ground rice cereal in place of cornmeal. It will be white but will taste terrific.

Yeast-Free White Bread

Finding a decent bread for sandwiches and toast is hard enough when you cannot use gluten, but add the yeast restriction and you really have problems. This bread mixes up quickly — it is really just a quick bread but resembles regular bread. It is certainly better than any yeast-free, GF bread you can buy, and it is easy to make.

1 Preheat oven to 350°F.

2 Spray an 8"×4" loaf pan with cooking spray, and coat with flour.

3 Combine flour, xanthan gum, baking powder, egg replacer, and salt in a bowl and mix with electric beater for approximately 30 seconds.

4 Combine eggs, water, oil, and honey in a bowl. Add to dry ingredients.

5 Mix on slow until well combined.

6 Pour batter into prepared pan and bake for 55–60 minutes. Test for doneness with a toothpick. The loaf should be golden on top and test dry in center.

Makes 1 medium loaf

2 cups GF flour mix

1 tablespoon xanthan gum

1 tablespoon GF baking powder

2 teaspoons egg replacer

1 teaspoon salt

2 eggs, slightly beaten

1 ⅓ cups water

2 tablespoons vegetable oil

1 tablespoon honey (optional, or use other sweetener such as pure vegetable glycerin)

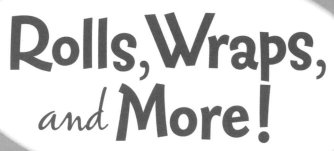

Rolls, Wraps, and More!

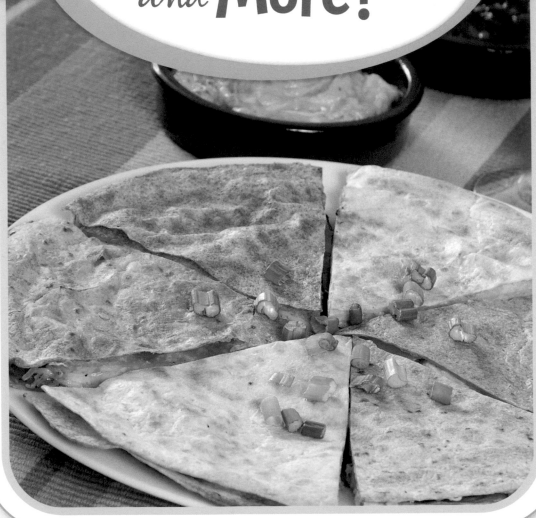

GFCF Tortillas/Wraps, recipe on page 84

Sweet Potato Rolls

These rolls are similar to biscuits. They make a nice mid-morning snack, or lunch filler. Do not be put off by the sweet potato — even children who do not like sweet potatoes will enjoy these rolls. They rise very little, so make the rounds at least ½" thick. They are a great addition to a holiday table.

1 Preheat oven to 450°F.
2 Steam or microwave potato until tender, but not mushy.
3 Blend until smooth in food processor or blender.
4 Measure potato puree — you will need 1 cup — and chill for 10-15 minutes.
5 Blend (or process) the potato, along with nut butter, juice, and maple syrup, until smooth.
6 Sift together flours, xanthan gum, baking powder, baking soda, and cardamom in a bowl, then work into the potato mixture by hand.
7 Form dough into a ball and roll out on a GF flour–covered surface. The dough will be smooth, pliable, and easy to roll out.
8 Roll out to ½" thickness and cut out rolls with a biscuit cutter or the rim of a drinking glass.
9 Bake on oiled or sprayed cookie sheets at 15 minutes, or until golden.

Makes 6 rolls

1 large sweet potato, peeled and diced
¼ cup nut butter, smooth
¼ cup pear juice
3 tablespoons pure maple syrup
1¼ cups GF flour
¾ cup brown rice flour
2 teaspoons xanthan gum
2 teaspoons GF baking powder
½ teaspoon GF baking soda
¼ teaspoon ground cardamom*

* You may use 1 teaspoon cinnamon in place of cardamom.

Mini Sandwich Rolls

½ cup oil

½ cup milk substitute

½ cup tapioca starch flour

½ cup potato starch

½ cup quinoa or chickpea flour

1 tablespoon sugar

1 tablespoon Ener-G egg replacer, plus amount liquid suggested (or 1 egg)

2 teaspoons xanthan gum

2 teaspoons GF baking powder

These rolls contain no gluten, rice, dairy, egg, or yeast. It is a wonder they are so good! If they are made into large rolls, they can be used for hamburger buns. Smaller ones toast nicely for breakfast or lunch.

1 Preheat oven to 400°F.

2 Beat together oil and milk substitute in a bowl.

3 In a separate bowl, mix starches, flour, sugar, egg replacer, xanthan gum, and baking powder.

4 Add liquid mixture to dry mixture and combine until just mixed. Do not overmix.

5 Spoon batter into ungreased muffin tin, or spoon onto a cookie sheet.

6 Bake for about 20–25 minutes or until golden brown. Do not crowd them as they puff up quite a bit.

7 Store in airtight container, or freeze.

Makes 12 rolls

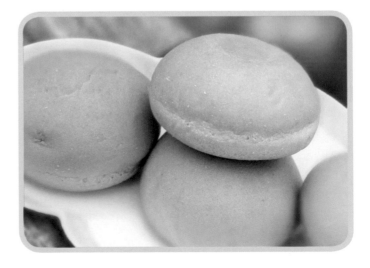

Porridge with a Purpose

Many come to the GFCF diet because of GI problems — in short, their children are constipated! Often parents believe that the opposite is their problem, but Drs. Simon Murch and Andrew Wakefield (Wakefield, et al., 2000) have shown that children with autism who seem to have diarrhea often are so constipated that an abdominal X-ray reveals impacted feces. What seems to be diarrhea is the liquid portion that can get around the impaction. Yuck. Not a pretty picture.

For all these children it is important to promote and maintain what the commercials call "regularity." Here is a recipe that will help. High in fiber and nutritious essential fatty acids, this hot cereal should be a "regular" on your breakfast table.

1 Bring water and salt to a boil and stir in cereal.
2 Cook over low heat for 1 minute, stirring constantly.
3 Remove from heat and stir in flax seed, cinnamon, and sweetener. Add dried fruit if desired.
4 Stir in enough milk substitute to reach desired consistency and serve.

Servings will vary.

1 cup water
Dash of salt
2 tablespoons GF hot cereal, uncooked (e.g., Cream of Rice)
2 tablespoons ground flaxseed or Nutriflax powder
½ teaspoon cinnamon
Sugar or other sweetener, to taste
Raisins or other dried fruit (optional)
DariFree™ or other milk substitute

GFCF Tortillas/Wraps

2 tablespoons shortening
   (Crisco or CF margarine)
2 cups Gluten-Free Pantry
   French Bread/Pizza Mix
1 teaspoon baking powder
½ teaspoon xanthan gum
½ cup hot water

Many Mexican recipes call for the use of soft flour tortillas, and in the last few years everyone has gone "wrap crazy." Many restaurants serve their most popular sandwiches in wrap-form — even that place with the golden arches! Soft wraps are great for sandwiches, and they also make a great breakfast wrap; fill it with scrambled eggs or breakfast meat, and you have an easy to eat, easy to carry morning meal.

Gluten-Free Pantry customer Elaine Smith developed a recipe for tortillas using the French Bread/Pizza Mix sold by the company. This recipe will not work with regular GF flour — the tortillas become very dry and break when you roll them out, but Gluten Free Pantry products are now widely available in grocery stores, and online at www.glutenfree.com.

Brown rice tortillas are available from Food For Life. Many health food stores and specialty markets, such as Whole Foods, carry them (look in the freezer section). They are best when slightly heated as they are a bit "stiff" when at room temperature.

1 Cut shortening into remaining ingredients (except water) until crumbly in a bowl. Mixture should resemble a pie crust.
2 Add water to dry ingredients and mix until a smooth ball is formed.
3 Invert on a lightly (rice) floured work surface and let rest 5 minutes.
4 Pinch off golf ball–sized pieces of dough. Roll out the pieces into circles 6–8" in diameter.

5 Heat an ungreased griddle to high.

6 Place tortillas on griddle and bake just until a bubble appears in the center of the tortilla. Flip over and cook just until done, less than 1 minute.

7 These can be frozen and reheated on a hot griddle or frying pan, but do not reheat well in a microwave.

Makes 10–12 tortillas

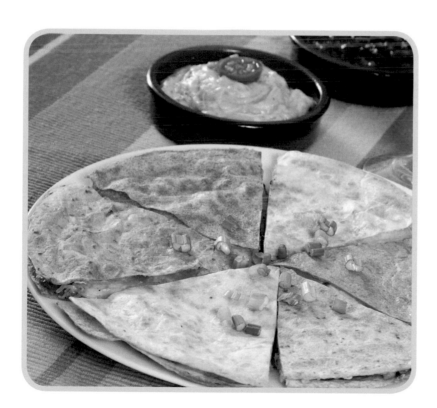

Breakfast Cookies

Liquid Ingredients

1 stick CF margarine, softened

⅓ cup pure maple syrup
   or honey*

1 egg

½ cup orange juice*

1½ teaspoons vanilla extract

Dry Ingredients

1 cup GF flour blend
   (I like Hagman's Four Flour
   Bean Mix)

1 cup GF oats or thinly sliced
   poha**

⅓ cup dry DariFree™

⅓ cup rice bran

1 tablespoon calcium powder
   (available from Kirkman
   Laboratories)

1 tablespoon Nutriflax powder
   (available at health
   food stores)

1½ teaspoons xanthan gum

1 teaspoon GF baking powder

1 teaspoon salt

1 cup raisins*
   (or other dried fruit)

⅓ cup pecans, ground
   (or other nuts, if tolerated)

¼ cup unsweetened coconut
   flakes (no sulfites)

These breakfast cookies pack a powerful nutrition punch. They have calcium (from the DariFree™ and calcium powder), protein (from the egg, pecans, and bean flour), iron (from raisins), and essential fatty acids (from the flax powder). They are not terribly sweet, and are easily modified for yeast-free regimens. I like this recipe so much that we featured it in *The ANDI News* and in *The Autism-Asperger's Digest Magazine*. Do not be put off by the long list of ingredients — they are easy to make. I have modified it slightly from the original version.

1 Preheat oven to 350°F.

2 Spray 2 cookie sheets with cooking spray.

3 Cream together margarine and maple syrup in a large bowl. Beat in egg. Add juice and vanilla.

4 Add dry ingredients except for raisins, nuts, nd coconut. Mix well.

5 Stir raisins, nuts, and coconut into the mixture.

6 Drop cookies on greased cookie sheet, 2" apart.

7 Bake 10–12 minutes.

Makes 24 cookies

*If you are avoiding yeast, you can use 100% pure vegetable glycerin flavored with GF maple flavoring instead of maple syrup. This very sweet liquid does not feed yeast. Squeeze fresh orange juice immediately before making the cookies to avoid any fermentation (often a problem with juices made from concentrate, or that have been in the refrigerator for any period of time). Omit dried fruit.

**Oats do not contain gluten, but most are contaminated with other grains and cannot be trusted. There is a company that "guarantees" that their oats are uncontaminated and thus truly gluten-free, but they are also quite expensive. If you want to give them a try, you can order online at www.glutenfreeoats.com. If you prefer, you can generally find poha, which is available at Indian markets. Or you can substitute quinoa flakes. Quinoa flakes are available at most groceries, though they are very crunchy.

✹ Crêpes

3 eggs
1 cup milk substitute
½ cup potato starch
Oil
2 tablespoons ghee, melted
Pinch salt

My husband was born in France and still has friends and relatives there. That is our excuse for visiting every few years, but we both love Paris so much that we would find another excuse if necessary! The first time we took our son Jacob with us, he was thrilled to discover the joy of standing at a window or cart, watching his very own crêpe spread out on the iron with the special little wooden rake. Then it was turned and, finally, spread with something delicious. I always tried to get him to save me just one bite, but it did not happen often. Luckily crêpes are also extremely versatile — they can be filled with savory foods for lunch or dinner, fruit for breakfast or dessert, or used to hold a delicious, portable omelet or scrambled eggs. For the purist, a thin spread of nut butter and jam makes a delicious (and portable) breakfast.

1 Combine the eggs and milk substitute in a blender or food processor and then add the potato starch.
2 Chill mixture for 30 minutes.
3 Swipe the inside of a 9" skillet with oil, or use cooking spray.
4 Place the pan on medium heat.
5 While the pan is heating, whisk the ghee into the chilled crêpe mixture.
6 Ladle in about 2 tablespoons batter, and turn the pan until the bottom is coated with batter. Remember, you want the crêpes to be thinner than American-style pancakes.

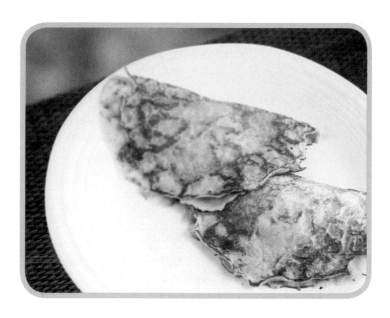

7 Cook crêpes for about 1 minute. When it looks dry, lift the edge with a small spatula and flip it over. (I lift the edge with an icing knife and then flip it with my fingers, but if you do this take care not to burn yourself.) The second side should cook in 30 seconds.

8 Remove to a plate and repeat until the batter is used. Spray the pan or wipe with oil before you make each crêpe.

Servings will vary.

CHAPTER 5

Drinks

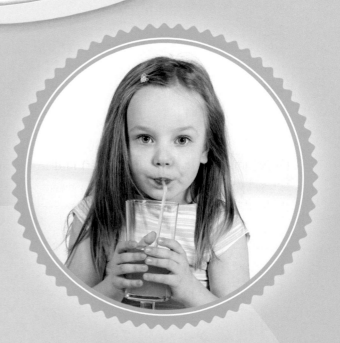

A lot of things have changed since I wrote the first volume of *Special Diets for Special Kids*, but one thing that has remained the same is that American children drink too much juice. The juice container may tout "no added sugar," and the juice within may be fortified with vitamins, but fruit juice is still pretty much all sugar. Juice has few nutrients, no fiber, and it takes up room in tiny tummies that should be saved for nutritious foods and drinks.

Dr. Richard Johnson and Timothy Gower (2008) implicate fructose (fruit sugar) in diabetes, hypertension, and obesity in a recent study; this link between disease and fructose appears to be only from juices, which contain highly concentrated amounts of the sugar. Whole fruits do not seem to correlate with these diseases. When a child is thirsty, we should encourage them to drink water or other drinks that do have some nutritional benefits.

Kids love their juice though, so we should aim for turning these nutritional lemons into lemonade whenever possible. One way to do this is to make sure that our drinks are as low in sugar as possible, and to use drinks made from the whole fruit whenever possible. We can also add sources of protein, calcium, and vitamins. We can even get fiber into a drink if we make it the right way.

I'm often asked whether or not someone needs to buy a particular cooking implement or appliance, and in general I do not believe you need a lot of "fancy stuff" to cook good, healthful meals. I do believe, however, that an investment in a really top-notch blender will pay off in the end.

I use a Vitamix 5200, and there are other similar machines on the market. These powerful blenders allow you to make everything from soup and nut butter to frozen desserts and, of course, smoothies. Using my Vitamix, I can whip up a frozen dessert in 5 minutes, and it allows me to add vegetables to food that will not will not will not be discernible to even the pickiest child! Unlike a typical juicer, it allows you to use the whole fruit, adding nutrients and fiber to the diet in a form all children love. It is my "go-to" appliance for healthful drinks, and even though it takes up valuable counter real estate, it is always plugged in and ready to go.

If you have a decent blender and a food processor, you might be able to duplicate some of the action of a high-end blender, but you will need to work in smaller batches and will likely need to strain the final product. However, if you can afford it, I do recommend you purchase a high-end blender for your kitchen. Often you can find a good price on eBay or at Costco, and Vitamix sells reconditioned models with full warranties. If it is totally out of reach, I suggest you put one on your holiday wish list. Nearly everyone reading this book has at least one family member or friend who always wants to help but does not know how — this would be a great way for them to do something for your family! ★

When I first wrote *Special Diets*, the selection of liquid milk substitutes was limited. There was rice milk and soy milk, but that was about it. Now almond milk, hemp milk, coconut milk, and others have been added to the available choices. Any of these recipes will work with any of these substitutes, so use the one that works best for your child.

Note: When milk substitute powder is called for, the recipe will specify "powdered milk substitute" or "dry DariFree™" (if DariFree™ works better than other powders for that recipe). If you prefer to use a powdered soy milk substitute, that will work too. When liquid milk substitute is called for, the recipe will generally state only "milk substitute." In the recipes that follow, substituting sparkling mineral water for seltzer will add additional calcium.

Homemade Nut Milk

new

What? What kind of crazy person (nut) would make their own nut milk? That is what I used to think too, until I watched a YouTube video and decided to give it a shot. I was amazed ... what I made was white, creamy, and absolutely delicious. Some nuts have their own natural sweetness and need nothing at all added, and for others, a few chopped dates adds just the right touch. A few spoonfuls of calcium powder blended in makes it even better.

To make your own nut milk, you only need four things: nuts, water, a fine mesh bag (a nut milk bag), and a blender. If you cannot find a nut milk bag (they are available online and in some health food stores), you can head over to Home Depot's paint department — the paint straining bags are almost identical to the fancy nut milk bags, and probably cost a lot less.

To watch the video that inspired me to make nut milk, go to www.purejoyplanet.com.

1 Place nuts and vanilla in a blender. Add water and dates or sweetener. Blend until the rattling noise stops. (If you over-blend, the fiber from the nuts will block the holes of the bag, so be sure to stop when the rattling stops.)
2 Place a nut milk bag in a bowl, and gently pour the contents of the blender into the bag. Pull the drawstring to close, then lift the bag, being careful not to miss the bowl. Gently "milk" the bag, squeezing gently until you have gotten all the liquid squeezed out.

Makes 3 drinks

1 cup nuts and/or seeds*
  (e.g., add a handful of
  sesame seeds to 1 cup
  cashews)
1 teaspoon vanilla extract
  (or extract of choice)
2 cups water
  (amount of water is always
  double amount of nuts)
3–4 chopped dates or 2–3
  tablespoons honey or pure
  maple syrup (optional)

If using brown-skinned nuts, such as pecans or almonds, soak them overnight and then rinse until the water runs clear.

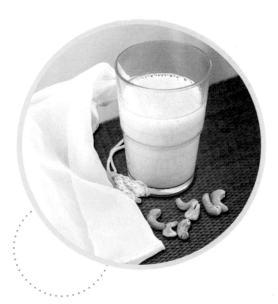

✳ *new* Rice Milk

4 cups water

1 cup cooked rice (brown is
    more nutritious)

1 tablespoon brown or
    turbinado sugar or 2–3 dates
    (optional)

1 tablespoon vanilla extract
    (optional)

Rice milk is widely available, but most brands are high in sugar. Since it is easy to make at home, especially with a high-end blender, it seems a shame to spend all that money on it. What a great way to use up leftover rice!

1 Place all ingredients in a blender and blend until desired consistency is reached. If you do not have a powerful blender, you will have to strain the milk.

2 Store milk in the refrigerator and shake before using.

Makes 4 drinks

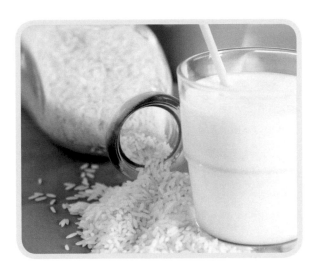

Kiddie Colada

This is a tasty, refreshing treat that most children will love. If possible, use fresh fruit. If you do not have a high-powered blender, you may need to strain before serving, but with a good blender this will not be necessary. Pineapple contains bromelain, a natural digestive enzyme, and has many vitamins. Bananas are high in potassium.

1 Combine all ingredients in a blender and process until you have a thick beverage.

Makes 2 drinks

I cup fresh pineapple chunks,
   plus ½ cup water (or 2
   (6-ounce) cans unsweetened
   pineapple juice)
2 bananas
8 ounces coconut milk
   (not coconut "cream")
Several ice cubes

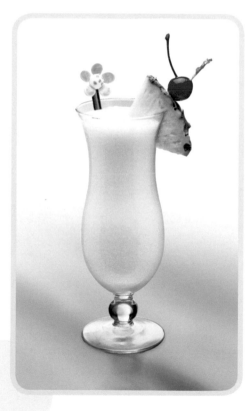

Mock Orange Julius

1 cup orange juice
  (preferably calcium fortified)
1 cup water
1 heaping cup ice
¼ cup sugar or sugar
  substitute
¼ cup dry DariFree™
2 tablespoons dehydrated egg
  white (e.g., Just Whites)
¼ teaspoon calcium powder

I have never really enjoyed malls, but I do have fond memories of those delicious orange drinks. This non-dairy recipe is very similar to the drink I remember. If your child cannot tolerate citrus, try using unsweetened pineapple juice or a fruit nectar.

1 Blend all ingredients in a blender or food processor on high for 30 seconds, or until drink is thick and smooth.

Makes 2 drinks

✴ Blueberry Shake

Adding calcium powder really boosts the nutritional value of this shake. To add protein, add 2 teaspoons dehydrated egg white or some tofu (if soy is tolerated).

I Puree the fruit in your blender, and then add the remaining ingredients. Blend until smooth. If it is too thick, add a little more water.

Makes 2 drinks

> **Hint:** If you use frozen fruit, you will not need ice to make a thick shake. If using frozen fruit, put all the ingredients in at the same time.

I ripe banana

I cup blueberries

2 cups ice, crushed

¼ cup dry DariFree™ or other powdered milk substitute

¼ cup milk substitute or water

I teaspoon calcium powder (optional)

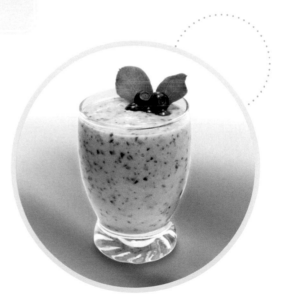

Fruit Smoothies

Shakes and smoothies make a good lunch for a little one who does not sit still long enough to eat a full lunch because you can easily hide a lot of nutrients in them. They are also great for breakfast because they can be whipped up in an instant and are easily portable. They make good desserts, and leftovers can be frozen into "ice cream" pops.

Using my Vitamix, I make all my smoothies the same way. I blend frozen fruit, preferably organic, and juice or milk substitute. If the fruit is not frozen, you can add a few ice cubes, but the product is creamier and nicer if you use frozen fruit. If I am in the mood, I also add some CF yogurt.

The bottom line is that making smoothies is not rocket science! Whatever combination of fruit, juice, or "milk" that your family likes will probably make a great drink. Just remember that very sweet fruit will require little sweetening. If needed, add a little sugar or honey to taste, or blend in a few chopped dates.

Hint: *When a banana or peach starts to get too ripe, peel it and freeze. I always have some frozen bananas on hand because they are fantastic to throw into drinks and desserts, and they thicken smoothies beautifully. Fruits are much harder to peel when they are frozen, so be sure to peel first. In summer, when blueberries are in season, be sure to freeze them too. Place berries on a cookie sheet, not touching each other, and freeze for 30 minutes. Bag the berries and put back in the freezer.*

Here are a couple smoothie suggestions to get you started. ★

World's Easiest Fruit Smoothie

This really is an easy thing to whip up and it is delicious. If you are following a restricted carbohydrate diet like the SCD, you will need to make your own almond milk since store brands contain starches. (See Homemade Nut Milk recipe on page 93.)

1 Put all ingredients in a blender and let it rip! Blend until smooth.

Makes 2 smoothies

I cup unsweetened berries, frozen (one type or a combination)
I cup unsweetened almond milk
2 teaspoons honey (or to taste)
I teaspoon vanilla extract (optional)*

If you use unsweetened vanilla almond milk, you can omit the vanilla extract.

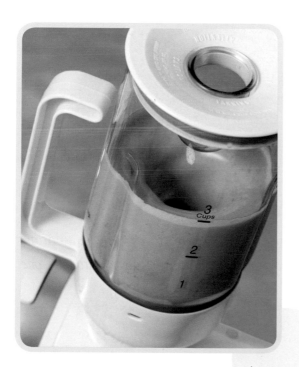

✳ new Mixed Berry Smoothie

1 cup cranberry juice or
   pomegranate juice
1 cup raspberries, frozen
½ cup blueberries, frozen
12 strawberries, frozen
1–2 bananas, frozen
1 teaspoon calcium powder
   (optional)

1 Blend all ingredients in a blender until smooth.

Makes 2 smoothies

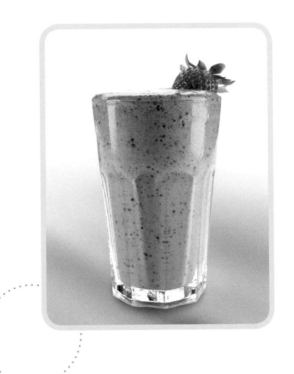

✳️ Green Smoothie

If you have a high-end blender, you can make this nutritious smoothie without straining, and you will be getting more nutrition and fiber. Most children will not eat kale, but when mixed with fruit, these veggies taste really good! If necessary, strain into a pitcher using a "nut milk bag" (a nut milk bag can be purchased from many health food stores or from Amazon.com for under $15) or a paint straining bag (available at home supply stores).

1 Add fruit, lemon juice, and kale to a blender. Add water to just below the top level of ingredients. Add stevia or other sweetener if desired. Blend to make a delicious green smoothie.

Makes 3–4 smoothies

1 orange, peeled with white
   pith removed
1 apple, seeded and cored but
   unpeeled
1 banana
3–4 chopped dates
1 tablespoon lemon juice
4–5 kale leaves
Water
Stevia or other sweetener
   (optional)

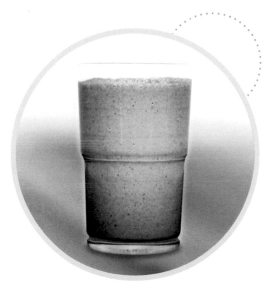

 Green Lemonade

6 organic kale leaves, stalk
  removed
1 organic lemon, unpeeled and
  quartered
6 stalks celery
1" knob of ginger root, peeled
1 apple, sliced but unpeeled
  (any variety)
1 tablespoon sugar or honey
  (optional)

Here's another "green" recipe because getting enough green vegetables in our children (and sometimes our significant others) is always a challenge. Most children do not like salad and even adults get tired of eating greens. Filled with vitamins and minerals, this one also packs an antioxidant punch. If you are not using a powerful blender, peel the lemon. When you are using a whole fruit, be sure to use organic when possible, and always wash it carefully. If you are using a food processor or less powerful blender, strain before serving.

1 Blend all ingredients in a blender until well blended. Sweeten with sugar or honey if desired.

Makes 2 drinks

★ Purple People Pleaser

This smoothie is "green" in that it contains spinach and kale, but when you pour it you will understand the name! It is actually purple and sure to delight most kids.

I Blend pineapple, blueberries, and water in a blender. Then add the greens. Taste to make sure you have not gone "too green" for your kids — in other words, you want it to taste fruity and not leafy. If it is too green, add more pineapple to taste. Blend well so there are not chunks or visible leaves. For less powerful blenders, make in smaller batches and strain if necessary. If your fruit is sweet, you should not need to add honey or dates, but you can if desired.

Makes 3 drinks

2 cups fresh pineapple, cored if
   not using a powerful blender
I cup blueberries
½ cup water
2 kale leaves, stalk removed
Spinach (add by handfuls
   and taste)
I tablespoon honey or 2–3
   dates (optional)

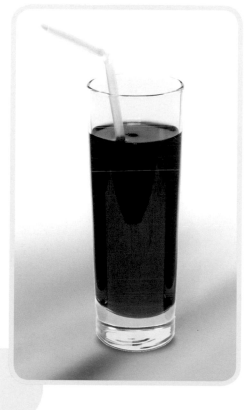

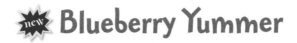 Blueberry Yummer

1 cup watermelon

1 cup blueberries, frozen

1 banana, frozen

½ avocado

1 lemon, juiced

4 kale leaves, stalk removed

If you have ever attended an Autism Research Institute conference, you have probably seen or met my friend Charlie Fall. At a smidge over 6 feet and with a delightful English accent, she can be hard to miss. Charlie is also an excellent and inventive cook, and she is a nutritional consultant to parents using biomedical interventions. Like me, Charlie is devoted to her Vitamix and is always coming up with great ways to use it. This recipe was made using leftovers, and the avocado will add creaminess (without adding a "green" taste). In addition, avocados act as a "nutrient booster," enabling the body to absorb more fat-soluble nutrients, such as alpha- and beta-carotene and lutein, in foods that are eaten with the fruit. By the way, this too will be purple.

1 Blend all ingredients in a blender and enjoy! Note that the watermelon adds so much liquid that additional water or juice is not needed…ingenious!

Makes 2 drinks

Mango Lassi

A *lassi* is a traditional Indian drink that may have been the original smoothie! They are often on the menu at Indian restaurants, but are always made with dairy. A delicious lassi can be made using CF ingredients, too. While mango is the most traditional flavor, use peach or other flavors if your children prefer.

I Blend all ingredients in a blender to make a thick lassi. You can add ice if you like it very thick.

Makes I drink

½ cup mango chunks, frozen (available at Trader Joe's and other groceries)
½ cup milk substitute
½ cup CF yogurt, plain (I prefer So Delicious coconut yogurt)
I tablespoon sugar or other sweetener
½ teaspoon cardamom (optional, but traditional)
Ice (optional)

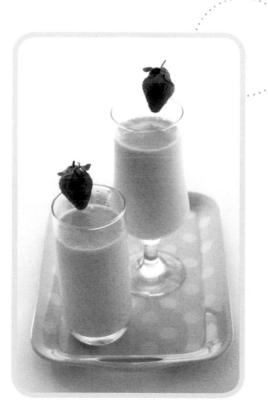

New York Egg Cream

¼ cup DariFree™ or other milk
  substitute
3 tablespoons chocolate syrup
6 ounces seltzer
  (or sparkling mineral water
  that contains calcium, such
  as Gerolsteiner)

The first night I spent as a New Yorker, I was squired around and treated to dozens of typical New York delicacies. Egg cream was one of them. As a Midwesterner, I found this drink puzzling — no eggs, no cream. Every New Yorker has his or her ideas about what makes it "authentic." Because this recipe is dairy-free, I do not claim it as a "real" egg cream, but I do think your child will find it a special treat.

1 Combine milk substitute and chocolate syrup in the bottom of an 8-ounce glass, then fill with seltzer and stir.
2 Serve while fizzy.

Makes 1 drink

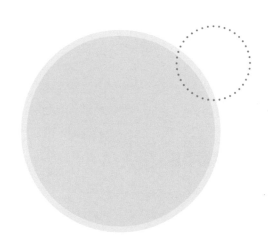

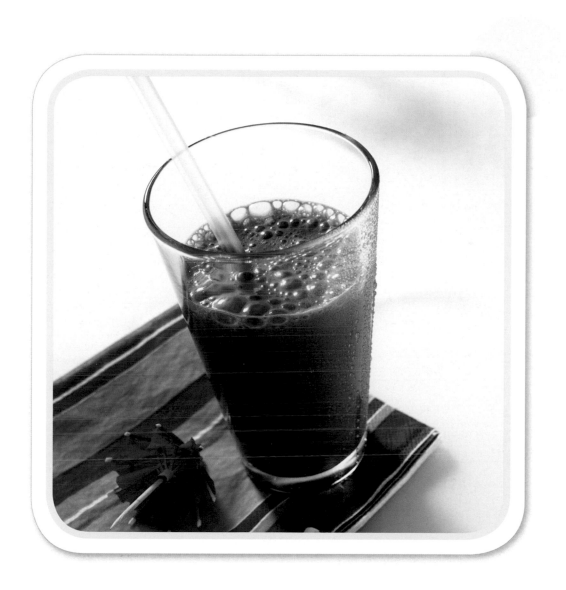

Other Drinks

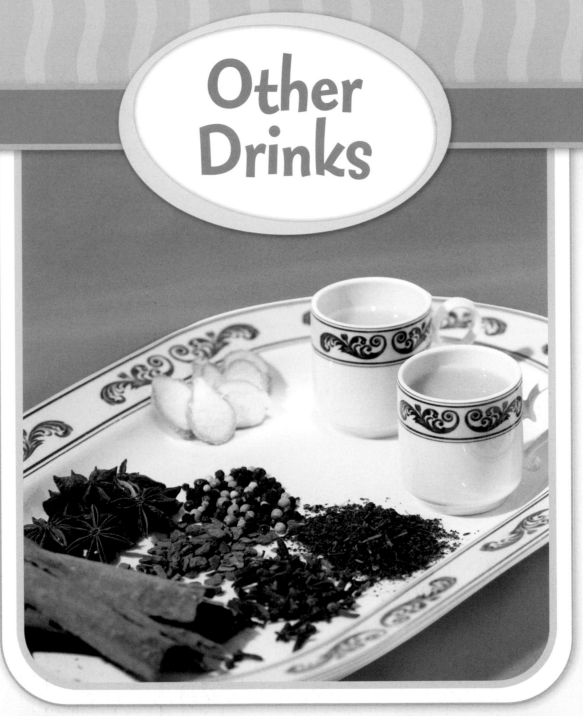

Chai, recipe on page 109

Chai

Chai is a word that, in much of the world, simply means tea. In the last few years, however, it has been used to describe a milky tea drink that is popular in coffee houses. It is easy to make your own, and it is a nice change of pace on a hot day. This recipe will make a powder that will keep indefinitely, and is mixed with the milk substitute of your choice.

Chai Powder

1 Grind all ingredients to a powder in a clean coffee grinder. Store in airtight container.

2 sticks cinnamon

3 whole cloves

5 cardamom pods
   (available in Indian markets)

1 peppercorn

1 allspice berry

1 teaspoon ground ginger

Chai

1 Bring water to a boil with sugar. Add chai powder. Mix well and remove from heat. Let the mixture "steep" for about 10 minutes.

2 Heat (but do not boil) milk substitute.

3 Pour ½ cup milk substitute into each of four glasses. Then pour 1 cup chai mixture into each cup. Pour through a strainer if desired. Mix well.

4 Chill before serving.

3 cups water

1 tablespoon sugar

4 teaspoons chai powder
   (see recipe above)

2 cups milk substitute

Makes 4 drinks

Variation: To make a frozen chai (such as found at many popular coffee restaurants), chill the prepared chai. Put in a blender with 1 cup ice and blend until cold and thick.

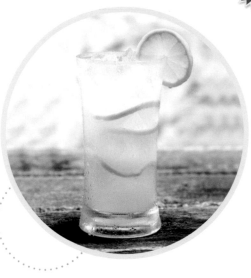

✸ new Lemonade: Three Ways

Lemonade is the summertime drink that everyone loves. The stuff you get at the grocery store, however, is filled with sugar or more likely, high fructose corn syrup. It usually has artificial colors and flavors, too. Since it is so easy to make (and to modify for special diets), why not do it yourself? If your children are used to commercially prepared lemonade, this might not seem sweet enough to them. You can add more sugar syrup, but gradually reduce it until you are using "just enough."

Traditional Lemonade

¼ cup sugar
¼ cup water
4 lemons
Water

1 Make a simple syrup by heating the water and sugar over medium heat until the sugar is completely dissolved.

2 Juice lemons and strain out any seeds, then pour into a large jar or pitcher. Add simple syrup and then enough water to make ½ gallon.

3 Stir or shake well, chill, and serve over ice. (When cold you can also freeze into ice pops.)

Makes ½ gallon (64 ounces) or 8 drinks

Variation: Add some frozen strawberries or raspberries to the simple syrup. It will be naturally pink and very tasty.

Charlie's Quick Lemonade

If desired, this sugar-free recipe can be doubled.

1 Stir lemon juice and water in pitcher and then add sweetener drop by drop, to taste. These sweeteners are one hundred times sweeter than sugar, so experiment to get the level of sweetener you prefer.

Makes 16 ounces or 2 drinks

2 lemons, juiced

16 ounces water

Stevia* liquid or xylitol syrup
   (to taste)

 Stevia is a herb found in liquid, powdered, or leaf form. It is much sweeter than sugar, so it is important to add it slowly and keep tasting. It does not raise blood sugar and does not feed yeast. The concentrated liquid version sold by Body Ecology does not have the licorice aftertaste common in stevia products. It can be purchased from Bodyecology.com or other online stores such as Amazon.com. Because it is so concentrated, a 2-ounce bottle will probably last for months!

Lemonade Soda

Using Gerolsteiner sparkling mineral water adds calcium and other minerals, and makes a fizzy version.

1 Mix all ingredients and serve over ice.

Makes 2 drinks

1 lemon, juiced

1 cup Gerolsteiner sparkling
   mineral water

1 cup spring water

Xylitol syrup or stevia (to taste)

Ice

Variation 1: Add a small pinch of sea salt for your own version of Gatorade.

Variation 2: Add grated ginger or ginger slices to 16 ounces boiling water, along with lemon juice. Chill and sweeten as desired.

Lunchtime!

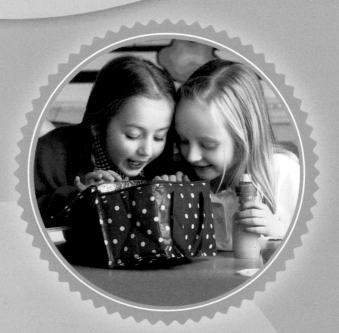

Lunch seems to be a hard meal for parents of children on special diets. It is easy to see why, since most people think "sandwich" when they think lunch. When we have to send lunch to school, a sandwich is the easiest, most portable thing most of us can think of. But not all our special breads hold up so well for sandwiches, and if you are trying to reduce the carbohydrates your children are eating, sandwiches are not a very good choice.

When my children were little, I noticed that they *dissected* most sandwiches before eating. Usually they would take it completely apart and eat the meat or other filling. Then they would eat their fruit, and if they were not too full, they would eat the bread. It occurred to me that for them at least, the bread really was just filler.

I bought them each a thermal food jar and started sending hot lunches. They learned to eat (and enjoy) soups, chili, stuffed spuds, stews, and their favorite leftover dinners at lunchtime. I would heat the food up while they ate breakfast, and by lunchtime the food had cooled to just the right temperature. The only hard part was getting them to remember to bring the food jar home, but with the help of teachers and paraprofessionals, they managed to remember most days.

I highly recommend getting a couple of these food jars. Thermos makes unbreakable versions (no glass) with kid-friendly designs. The jar will keep food cold, too, so you could send in any cold salads or other foods that your child likes.

If your child prefers breakfast to other meals, you can use these foods to make a nutritious lunch that will actually be eaten. Mini muffins or muffin tops are great lunch-box additions, and can serve as a nutritious "dessert." If your child loves waffles but hates GF bread, you can use them for sandwiches. Some children love leftover pancakes — if yours does, make extra the next time you make a pancake breakfast. The next day, spread a little nut butter and perhaps some jam on 2 or 3 pancakes, and roll them up tightly. If they will not stay rolled, use a toothpick to hold them together. They are fun to eat and nutritious.

When considering what to do about school lunches, take a minute to study the ubiquitous "Lunchable" in your store's refrigerator case. These ready-made school lunches are low on nutrition and high on price, but children love them. Why? Obviously, the trick is in the packaging. Another thing that attracts children is that the foods are in appropriately small servings (we tend to give our children adult portions). If you think your child would find it appealing, create your own Lunchable, cutting GFCF lunchmeats into cubes or small circles. Add just two GF crackers, not a whole stack. Include a fruit and a few carrot sticks if your child likes crunch. Add two small cookies or a mini muffin, and you have a lunch your child might actually eat. After all, it does not matter how nutritious a meal is if it gets thrown away!

You can even pack lunch in a divided container to create your own (reusable) Lunchable. Tupperware makes a "Lunch N Things" container with four sections and a hinged top. It is like a reusable bento box for kids!

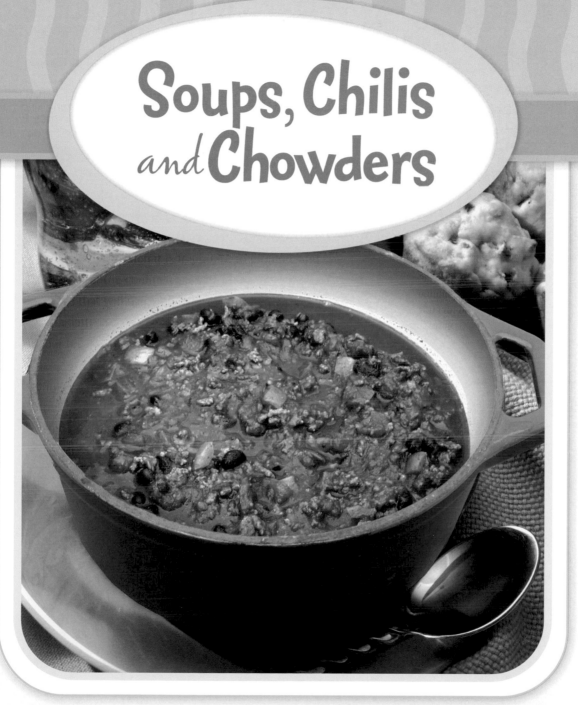

Soups, Chilis and Chowders

The World's Easiest Chili, recipe on page 121

Chicken Rice Soup

6 cups GF chicken broth

1 cup cooked chicken, diced

½ cup celery, chopped

1 carrot, chopped

1 small potato, peeled and
   diced

½ teaspoon dried parsley

Salt and pepper (to taste)

3 ounces long grain white rice,
   uncooked

Even really young children like chicken rice soup. There is no reason it has to come from a can, which can be pretty sorry stuff. Canned soups often contain many additives and preservatives, too. If you have homemade chicken broth, this soup is even more delicious, but a good GF canned broth will save time and energy.

1 Bring chicken broth to a boil in a large pot.

2 Add remaining ingredients (except rice), and return soup to a boil.

3 Lower heat, cover, and simmer for 10 minutes.

4 Add rice, stir, and simmer for 15–20 minutes, or until rice is tender.

Makes 4 servings

Lentil Soup

When Sam was about eight years old, he found that he loved soup. If asked what he wants for dinner, invariably he asks for chili, black bean, or lentil soup. Many parents do not introduce soups to their children, assuming that they will not eat them. Remember, most young children do not like very hot foods, but if the temperature is very warm but not hot, many will eat and enjoy soups. Because most soups can be pureed in a blender or food processor, they are also great for children with texture sensitivities. And do not forget to hide the veggies! If needed, puree the vegetables before adding them to the pot.

1 Combine broth, water, onion, celery, garlic, spaghetti sauce, and herbs in a large pot. Bring to a boil.

2 Rinse lentils under cold water and drain. Add lentils to pot.

3 Return pot to boiling, then lower heat.

4 Cover pot and let simmer for 30 minutes.

5 Add pasta. Bring to a boil and stir.

6 Lower heat and simmer for 30 minutes, stirring often. If soup becomes too thick, add a little more water.

7 Remove and discard bay leaf, season with salt and pepper, and serve.

Makes 4 servings

2 cups GF beef broth (or use water and GF bouillon)

6 cups water

1 medium onion, chopped

½ cup celery, chopped

¼ cup GF spaghetti sauce

2 garlic cloves, minced

1 bay leaf

1 tablespoon fresh parsley, chopped (or 1 teaspoon dried parsley)

½ teaspoon dried thyme

1 cup dry lentils

1 (3-ounce) package GF pasta

Salt and freshly ground black pepper (to taste)

 Note: *If you prefer, you can substitute ½ cup rice for pasta, or omit it entirely.*

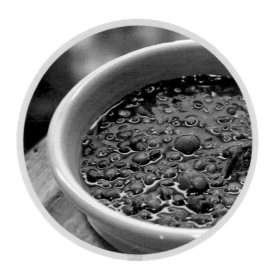

Red Lentil Soup (Dahl)

1 pound red lentils

3 tablespoons olive oil
  (or ghee)

2 onions, sliced thinly

4 garlic cloves, chopped

2 teaspoons fresh ginger,
  finely grated

6 cups hot water

1 teaspoon ground turmeric

2 teaspoons sea salt

1 teaspoon garam masala*

*Garam masala is an
Indian spice mixture that
can be bought in Indian
markets.*

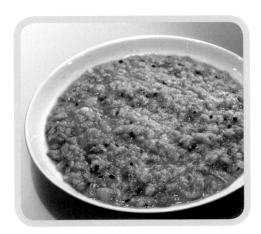

Our grocery stores often have just one kind of lentil — brown. My husband did fieldwork in Pakistan during the 1980s, and he says that there are literally hundreds of different pulses (lentils) available there. If you venture into an Indian shop, in this country you will not find hundreds, but you can find dozens of different lentils. Red lentils make an especially good soup because they cook very quickly into a thick, porridge-like consistency. They are also pretty, and very tasty. This is so easy; you may find yourself making it often. It works well with yellow lentils, too, though they take a little longer to cook.

1 Wash lentils in a large bowl, and throw away any that float to surface of water. Drain lentils and set aside.

2 Heat oil in a soup pot, and cook onions, garlic, and ginger until onions start to brown.

3 Stir in lentils, then add water. Bring to a boil, and then reduce heat.

4 Cover and cook over low heat for 30 minutes, stirring occasionally (be careful so lentils do not burn).

5 Stir in spices. Remove lid and cook until soup reaches consistency you want. If you want it very thick, leave lid off and cook until some of liquid evaporates. For thinner soup, omit this step.

6 You can also cook this into a very thick porridge and serve with rice as a main dish. It is high in protein.

Makes 4 servings

✳ Split Pea Soup

Split pea soup could not be easier — if you can boil water, you can make split pea soup! It freezes beautifully, so it is worth making 1 pound of peas at a time. Note that when it is stored, it will get very thick; because you add water or broth to thin it when you reheat the soup, it seems to last and last. Many people cook the soup with ham hocks, but I prefer a vegan version. If you want to, add 1–2 rinsed ham hocks to the soup and discard when the soup is cooked. Sometimes I add some browned stew meat and call it "dinner."

1 (1-pound) bag green split peas, picked over for stones or debris
2½ cups water (or vegetable or chicken broth)
2 carrots, peeled and chopped
2 celery stalks, chopped
1 onion, chopped
Salt and pepper (to taste)

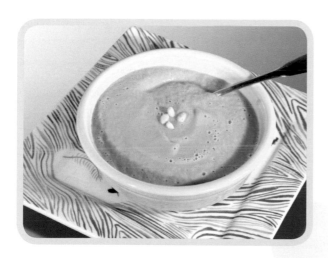

Chilled Almond Soup

¾ cup almonds, blanched

1 shallot (or small garlic clove)

3 tablespoons extra virgin
olive oil

¼ cup GF bread crumbs
(or GF panko) (optional)*

2 cups cold vegetable broth

Salt and pepper (to taste)

1 tablespoon apple cider
vinegar

Sliced almonds
(or green grapes)

 *The bread crumbs will thicken the soup, but can be left out with no effect on taste. Glutino now makes GF panko crumbs.

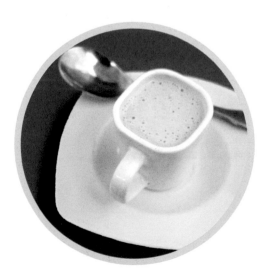

I saw this soup recipe on Salon.com and tracked down its author, Lucy Mercer. Lucy has a couple of terrific food blogs, and she was nice enough to let me include this yummy soup recipe. Its texture is velvety and lovely, and children will like eating it out of little cups. Sometimes called Ajo Blanco or White Gazpacho, it is simple, tasty, and kid-pleasing. It is also appropriate for those following the SCD (if you omit the optional crumbs). Check out Lucy's terrific recipes and interesting food commentary at http://acookandherbooks.blogspot.com. If you want to change it up and make a sweet soup, you can omit the onion and add 1 teaspoon honey.

1 Toast blanched almonds in a skillet for a few minutes, and remove from heat and let cool.

2 In a food processor or blender, purée shallot, then add toasted almonds. Blitz until finely ground. Add oil and bread crumbs, and process until combined.

3 With the motor running, slowly pour in broth through feed tube. Season with salt and pepper. Finish with cider vinegar.

4 Strain soup and serve in rimmed soup plates or demitasse cups, with a few sliced almonds or grapes for garnish. Lovely!

Makes 8 servings

The World's Easiest Chili

Most people think of chili as a winter dish, but my son does not believe in "seasonal" foods. (This also explains why I make cranberry sauce all year!) I used to make it in the traditional way, but sometimes you just need a shortcut. I found that by using a prepared salsa, I could make a terrific, super quick, and easy chili. Be sure to read the ingredients carefully when using prepared products like salsa. What I love about using salsa is that you can choose how hot or mild to make it, and how chunky you want it. My favorite salsa has black beans and corn, but there are many brands and styles available. We like it spicy, but feel free to walk on the mild side, especially if your family does not usually go for the hot stuff. Red kidney beans are traditional, but use whatever beans you like (or omit them entirely). I often use black beans or chickpeas.

1 Brown meat and drain off all fat. Add salsa and beans, bring to a simmer, and cook for 20 minutes.

2 Add salt and pepper to chili, and serve.

Makes 4 servings

Variation: Add some leftover rice for the last 5 minutes of cooking to make a hearty meal.

1 pound lean ground meat
(I use beef or turkey)
2 (16-ounce) jars salsa*
3 tablespoons chili powder
1 (15.5-ounce) can beans
(your choice), rinsed and
drained
Salt and pepper (to taste)

This makes a soupy consistency; if you like your chili thicker, use less salsa.

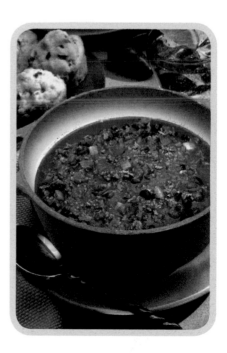

Chicken and Vegetable Chowder

6 bacon strips (nitrite-free)

I medium onion, diced

2 garlic cloves, minced

4 cups coconut milk

2 cups cooked chicken, diced

2 cups fresh corn*
   (or frozen corn)

2 cups fresh vegetables*
   (or frozen mixed vegetables)

I ½ cups mashed potato flakes
   (sulfite-free)

I (28-ounce) can GF chicken
   broth

I fresh basil sprig, chopped
   (or ½ teaspoon dried basil)

Salt and pepper (to taste)

 Fresh corn or other vegetables may be used. If your child will not eat anything recognizable as a vegetable, thaw and puree vegetables before adding them to pot.

I am not sure what makes a soup a chowder, but this is a good one no matter what you call it. If your child cannot eat corn, you can use other vegetables. Chowders are usually thickened with cream, but this recipe uses mashed potato flakes. Be sure to buy flakes that are sulfite- and additive-free (available at health food stores).

1 Cook bacon until crisp; reserve fat and set aside.

2 In stewpot or Dutch oven, cook onion and garlic in reserved fat. Onion should be soft but not browned.

3 Add remaining ingredients, and cook for 20 minutes over medium heat.

Makes 4 servings

Note: For vegetarian chowder, omit chicken broth and use vegetable broth instead.

Sandwiches, Rolls, and Wraps

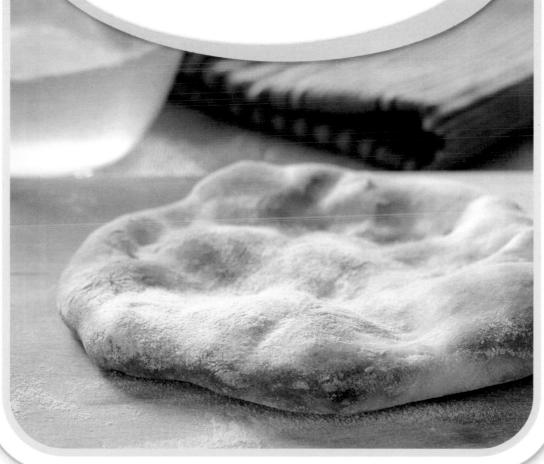

Buckwheat Pete's Honey-Buckwheat Pitas, recipe on page 126

PB and Peach Sandwich

GF bread or roll
   (particularly good with
   GF English muffins)
1 very ripe peach, peeled
Nut butter

If your child loves peanut butter and jelly, but is off sugar, try this slightly odd sandwich. My sister came up with the concept of a peach sandwich when she was on a very strict low-sugar diet. I know it sounds silly, but do not laugh until you have tried it. Children eat lots of things stranger than this. And of course, if your child cannot eat peanuts, there are dozens of other nut butters to try. If all nuts are off the table, try sesame paste (tahini).

1 Spread bread slice with nut butter, then top with peach. Top with another bread slice to create a sandwich.
2 If you want to make the peach more like jam, mash and drain it before topping the nut butter.

Makes 1 sandwich

Variation: A very ripe banana will also make a good PB and Fruit sandwich.

GF Spring Rolls

Most children like foods they can pick up and eat with their hands, and this recipe makes a great finger food. The filling is similar to a traditional egg roll, but you can use whatever your family enjoys and tolerates. Though this filling contains vegetables your child may not typically eat, do not be afraid to try it. Somehow, when veggies are wrapped in a spring roll, most children do like them. When buying spring roll wrappers, be sure you get the ones containing only rice and water (and perhaps salt). They will be round and brittle; the soft wrappers contain wheat flour. You will probably have to go to an Asian market for these, though I can often find them in the ethnic aisle of one of our larger supermarkets. These rolls are delicious and portable. Since they are good at room temperature, they are easy to wrap in foil and send as a school lunch.

Shredded cabbage
Mushrooms, chopped
GF broth
Canned bamboo shoots, chopped (optional)
Chopped onion (or scallion)
Cooked chicken, shredded
GF soy sauce
Garlic, minced
Ground ginger
Rice roll wrappers
Water

1 Preheat oven to 400°F.
2 Cook cabbage and mushrooms in a little broth. Then add remaining ingredients.
3 Cook until vegetables are soft and "sauce" thickens a bit to create filling.
4 Dip each wrapper separately in a bowl of hot water. It will soften in less than 1 minute.
5 Remove wrapper and add 2 tablespoons filling on top. Wrap up like an envelope, using water to seal edges if necessary.
6 Place rolls on a greased cookie sheet, and spray tops with vegetable spray.
7 Bake rolls for about 10 minutes, then turn and bake another 5 minutes, or until brown and crispy.

Servings will vary.

Note: It is tempting to fry these, but do not try it. The skins are too delicate to hold up to frying, and they will fall apart and leave you with a nasty, inedible mess. When baked, the rolls hold together and are very crispy.

Buckwheat Pete's Honey-Buckwheat Pitas

1½ cups light buckwheat flour
2 teaspoons dried chives
   (optional)
½ teaspoon salt
1 tablespoon honey
¼ cup sunflower oil
½ cup tapioca starch flour
1½ cups warm water

Peter de Niverville (aka "Buckwheat Pete") has published several e-books that can be purchased online, downloaded, and read or printed via Adobe Acrobat software. In the book, *Buckwheat Pete Bakes Pitas & Tea Biscuits*, Pete presents an unusual bread-making technique. It involves cooking tapioca starch flour until it is sticky and opaque, and then gently kneading it into the GF flour mixture. The cooked tapioca starch flour provides the binding and stretchiness that usually comes from xanthan or guar gum. Because xanthan gum is derived from corn, there may be some extremely sensitive people who cannot use it (though the vast majority can). Further, xanthan gum is very expensive and even though it is used in small amounts, it may be worth your while to experiment with Pete's method. Pete was kind enough to allow me to use his pita recipe, and I encourage you to visit Buckwheatpete.com for information on ordering his electronic books. For rice pitas, merely substitute white rice flour for buckwheat flour. These pitas form a strong pocket to stuff with your child's favorite sandwich filler.

1 Preheat oven to 375°F.
2 In a large mixing bowl, combine buckwheat flour, chives, and salt.
3 Add honey and oil, and blend with a pastry blender until mixture is grainy. Form a well in middle of flour mixture, and set aside.

4 Dissolve tapioca starch flour with water in a large, microwave-proof glass measuring cup. Microwave on high for 2–3 minutes, stirring twice, or until mixture has thickened and becomes clear and sticky. It should look like petroleum jelly, but will be thicker and stickier. There must be no liquid left in tapioca mixture, or tapioca will not bind with flour. Allow mixture to cool.

5 Place cooked tapioca in the well you made in flour mixture. Knead by hand until all flour has disappeared into mixture.*

6 Form dough into a ball. Divide the ball into 4 pieces, and form each into a patty.

7 On a GF-floured surface, roll out each patty to ⅛–¼" thickness. Use a spatula to transfer patties to a non-stick baking sheet.

8 Bake pitas for 15–18 minutes, or until slightly browned.

9 Put pitas on a wire rack to cool, and cover with a clean dishtowel.

Makes 4 servings

Kneading in all the flour mixture will take a little elbow grease, but do not give up. You will be rewarded with smooth, workable dough!

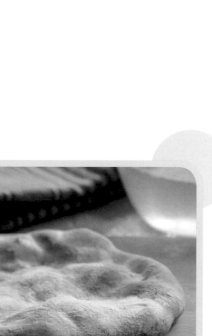

Potato Wraps

2 cups potatoes, mashed
1 cup GF flour
1 teaspoon salt
CF margarine, melted (or ghee)

I met Joya Sabouni after a speech I gave in Souderton, Pennsylvania. She has shared many of her inventive recipes over the years, including this one. This works well for wrap-type sandwiches. It is similar to a pita, and is a useful recipe for people who are using rotation diets.

1 Combine potatoes with flour and salt. Work together until it forms a dough.

2 Transfer dough to counter and shape into a long rope. Slice dough into 1" sections.

3 Roll slices of dough into round circles, the size of a tortilla or pita.

4 Heat a heavy, dry frying pan on top of a burner. When pan is very hot, put in a flatbread circle. Cook until dough blisters and begins to brown. Turn. Finish cooking other side. When all of them are done, brush with margarine.

5 Use like a pita or flatbread to wrap around your favorite filling.

Makes 4 servings

Meat and Potatoes

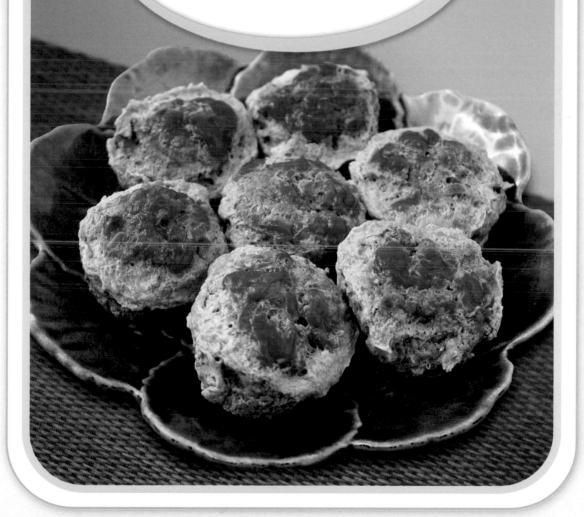

Meat (Loaf) Muffins, recipe on page 131

Meat Puffs

14 ounces meat (pork, turkey, or chicken), cooked

Water

½ cup GF breading,* ground finely in a food processor or coffee grinder

1 egg (or egg replacement substitute equivalent to 1 egg)

½ cup water (or milk substitute)

1½ teaspoons GF baking powder

Salt and pepper (to taste)

1 teaspoon flaxseed powder (optional)

¼–1 cup cooked vegetables, blended in a blender or food processor

Lisa Ackerman modified a recipe from *Special Diets for Special Kids* to make this tasty little item. Her son swears by it. She says that this recipe has helped even the fussiest children eat protein and veggies, and suggests starting with ¼ cup vegetables, then increasing to at least 1 cup over time. It is a good way to use up leftover meat.

1 Preheat oven to 350°F.

2 Puree meat with just enough water to make a paste.

3 Put all ingredients into bowl and mix well. Form meat mixture into little balls or logs.

4 Place balls on a lightly greased baking sheet.

5 Cook meat puffs for 18–25 minutes, or until light brown.

Makes 4 servings

*Lisa rotates her son's foods, so she uses quinoa flakes and quinoa flour one day, GF crispy rice cereal and rice flour on other days, and potato flour and potato buds on potato days. Allergy Grocer breading mix would be another good choice.

Meat (Loaf) Muffins

OK, so these are not really "muffins," but they look like muffins! Children often love individual portions, and may be happier to eat a meat loaf that comes as their own mini serving, rather than as a slice of the family's loaf. They are cute and easy to prepare, so give them a try. What is even better is that these cook in half the time of a regular meat loaf.

1 Preheat oven to 350°F.

2 Heat oil in a non-stick pan and cook onion, carrot, and garlic for a few minutes, until vegetables are soft. Set aside.

3 When onion mixture is cool, add it to ½ the tomato purée. Then mix in remaining ingredients.

4 Divide meat mixture between 12 cups of a greased muffin tin.

5 Top "muffins" with remaining tomato purée, about 2–3 teaspoons on each.

6 Bake meat muffins for 30 minutes.

7 Let stand for 10 minutes before serving.

Makes 12 servings

1 tablespoon olive oil

1 onion, finely chopped

1 carrot, grated

1 garlic clove, minced

1 cup tomato purée, divided

1½ pounds lean ground beef
   (or other ground meat)

½ teaspoon dried oregano

1 teaspoon honey (optional)

1 teaspoon GF Worcestershire
   sauce* (or soy sauce)

2 eggs

Salt and pepper (to taste)

 See recipe for Worcestershire sauce in chapter 11.

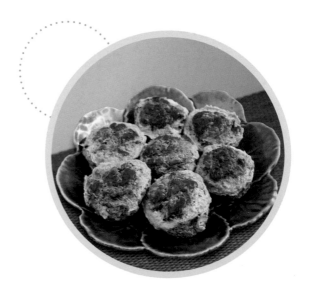

Potato Logs

4 large white potatoes, grated
and cooked

2 medium yellow squash,
grated but not cooked

¼ cup ghee, melted (or CF
margarine)

Sea salt and pepper (to taste)

Dedicated GFCF mom Lisa Ackerman contributed this recipe for potato logs, and promises your child will like them. If her son Jeff likes them, she is fairly sure that any kid will eat them. Lisa insists that he is the world's pickiest child, but then, I bet you think your child wins that award! Jeff gives this "two enthusiastic thumbs up."

1 Preheat oven to 425°F.

2 Combine potatoes, squash, and ghee in a bowl.

3 Season mixture with salt and pepper, and mix well. (Mixing with your hands may work best.)

4 Form mixture into little logs (no longer than the size of your palm), and place on ungreased cookie sheet.

5 Bake logs for 25 minutes, or until golden brown.

Makes 4 servings

Oven Fries

This is an easy way to cook "fries" if you are cutting back on fat. Some children will only eat potatoes that are actually fried, but most will accept oven-fried potatoes, too.

2 pounds potatoes
1 tablespoon oil (olive oil or safflower oil)
1 teaspoon imported sweet paprika
Sea salt (to taste)

1 Preheat oven to 425°F.

2 Wash potatoes well and peel, if you wish. In a large bowl, stir together oil and paprika. Set aside.

3 Cut potatoes lengthwise into ½" strips. Toss potatoes in oil-paprika mixture until well coated.

4 Arrange potatoes in a single layer on a lightly oiled baking sheet.

5 Bake 45–60 minutes, stirring occasionally, until fries are golden and crisp.

6 Sprinkle fries with salt and serve.

Makes 4 servings

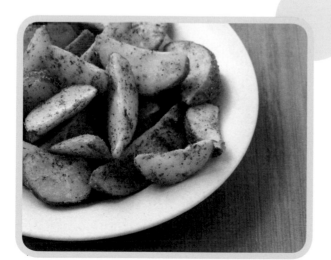

Other Lunchtime Favorites

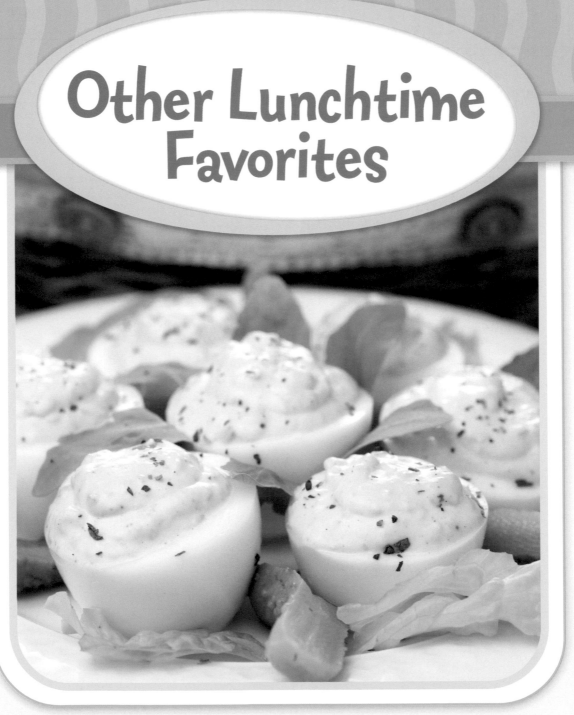

Deviled Eggs, recipe on page 135

Deviled Eggs

If eggs are tolerated, they are a terrific source of protein. Many children who would not dream of touching a plain egg will eat a deviled one. If you can, pipe the filling through a pastry tube. They look so appetizing when made this way that even a fussy little one may be induced to try them.

1 Cut eggs in half lengthwise. Remove yolks and set aside hard-boiled eggs.
2 Mash yolks with a fork, and mix with remaining ingredients.
3 Mound or pipe yolk mixture into hard-boiled eggs.
4 Sprinkle with paprika and serve.

Makes 12 servings

6 eggs, hard-boiled
¼ cup GFCF mayonnaise
½ teaspoon mustard
¼ teaspoon GF Worcestershire sauce
1 teaspoon sweet pickle relish (optional)
Salt and pepper (to taste)
Dash imported sweet paprika (optional)

Squash Latkes

1 spaghetti squash, cooked
   and removed from skin
   with a fork
2 eggs, beaten
Pinch salt
¼ cup GF cracker crumbs
   (or GF breading)
Oil

 Note: *Spaghetti squash has a pleasant, mild flavor. When it is served with marinara sauce, many children will eat it. You may also want to toss it with some CF margarine or a little melted ghee. Add salt and serve as a side dish.*

Latkes (pancakes) are traditionally made from potatoes. My friend Randee found herself with some extra spaghetti squash one summer, and got the bright idea of using it to make latkes. Her vegetable-phobic children had no idea what they were eating and gobbled them right down. You can cook the squash the night before, and store the "strings" in the refrigerator overnight. You could also substitute finely grated zucchini or yellow squash for the spaghetti squash.

1 Preheat oven to 375°F.
2 Pierce squash in several places, then place in a shallow pan.
3 Bake squash for 1 hour, until a fork can pierce easily.
4 When cool enough to handle, cut squash in half with a serrated knife. Scoop out seeds and fibrous strings from center of squash and discard.
5 Using tines of a fork, scrape out flesh of squash. It will come out in spaghetti-like strands.
6 Place squash in a large bowl and add eggs, salt, and enough cracker crumbs so that mixture is stiff enough to form into patties.
7 Heat oil for a few minutes, then form latkes with wet hands.
8 Fry latkes until golden and crispy on all sides.

Makes 4 servings

Crustless Quiche

This recipe makes a great breakfast or a light lunch. It is perfect to make ahead for those hectic school mornings, and great for those avoiding all starches and grains. You can also add chopped vegetables (¼ cup) if you want to. Be sure to use a natural bacon, without nitrites and other chemicals, but be aware that this bacon does not keep well and must be frozen. This quiche keeps well in the refrigerator if well wrapped.

6 bacon strips, cooked until crisp and blotted of excess fat
4 eggs
Approximately 1 cup milk substitute (see directions)
Salt and pepper (to taste)
Pinch ground nutmeg (optional)

1 Preheat oven to 350°F.
2 Crumble cooked bacon into bottom of an 8" pie or quiche pan.
3 Beat eggs in a 4-cup measuring cup, and add milk substitute to make 1½ cups total.
4 Season with salt, pepper, and nutmeg, and pour over bacon.
5 Bake for 30 minutes or until set.
6 Let quiche cool. Cut into wedges, wrap, and refrigerate.
7 Serve hot, warm, at room temperature, or chilled.

Makes 1 (8") quiche

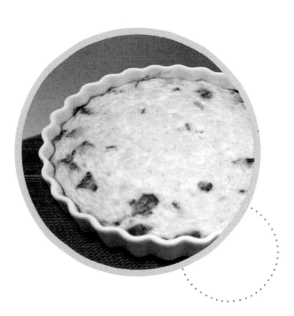

Variation: Add ½ cup Daiya "Cheese" Shreds to liquid mixture. Sprinkle a little Daiya on top before baking quiche.

Tamale Pie

Chili (vegetarian or chili
   con carne)
GF corn bread batter or sweet
   corn bread batter
   (see Mexican Corn Bread
   Pizza recipe on page 192)

Every chili lover knows that if there are any leftovers, Tamale Pie will make an appearance the next night! It is a great way to use up chili, and tasty enough to make even if you do not have leftovers. Use whatever amount of chili you like, depending on how many people the dish must feed. You may have to stretch the chili with some salsa or other ingredients.

1 Place chili in a 1- or 2-quart casserole, depending on amount you have.

2 Spoon ½ recipe of corn bread batter on top, and bake according to corn bread directions. (It is generally best to use only half the corn bread recipe for this dish — if you have too much batter on top, the corn bread sucks up all the liquid from the chili. It is still good, but in this case, less is more. Use other half of cornbread batter to make muffins or a mini loaf.)

Servings will vary.

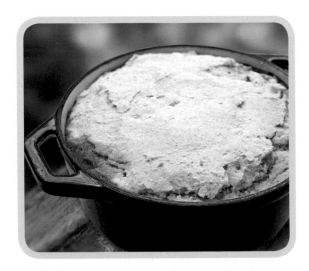

Asian Tenders

My son never tires of chicken tenders (or nuggets). Here is a slightly different take on them — one that your child will like if he or she enjoys the sweet dipping sauces available at some fast food restaurants. The sesame seeds add a nice flavor and a bit of calcium. If you prefer, these tenders can be fried.

1 Combine marmalade, ginger, garlic, and soy sauce in a baking pan (preferably glass).

2 Marinate and refrigerate chicken tenders in liquid mixture for at least 1 hour.

3 Preheat oven to 400°F.

4 Place sesame seeds in a dry skillet over medium heat, stirring often until they begin turning golden. Watch them carefully as they can burn quickly.

5 Cool seeds, and combine them with cereal in a pie pan or other low-sided dish.

6 Dip marinated tenders in cereal-seed mixture.

7 Bake tenders for 10 minutes, or until inside is not pink.

Makes 4 servings

¼ cup orange marmalade
(or pineapple marmalade)
½ teaspoon ground ginger
¼ teaspoon garlic powder
2 tablespoons GF soy sauce
(optional)
1 pound chicken tenders,
rinsed and dried*
¼ cup toasted sesame seeds
(optional)
3 cups GF crispy rice cereal,
lightly crushed

 It is much cheaper to buy chicken breasts and cut your own tenders. Just remove skin and visible fat, remove meat from bone and slice into desired size and shape. For thin tenders, place meat between sheets of wax paper and pound with a meat mallet. Baking time will vary, depending on how thin you slice tenders.

Anytime Snacks

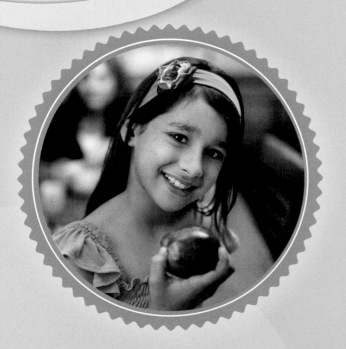

Children generally have small appetites, so they rarely eat a great deal at any meal. Most nutritionists suggest frequent small meals, rather than three square meals a day; that pattern certainly works best for young children. Preschoolers usually need a morning snack between breakfast and lunch, and at least one more snack before dinner.

School-aged children will head to the refrigerator as soon as they get home, and if they have a choice, they will fill up on junk. But snacks do not have to be just "empty calories," and they do not have to require a lot of fussing in the kitchen. While this chapter does give some recipes, I would like to make some general suggestions about how to handle snacktime.

Most importantly, think simple. Good snacks have few ingredients but lots of nutrients. They are not processed or refined, and they should be easy and quick to prepare. Think vitamins, fiber, flavor, and fun! The following are some examples of the easiest and most nutritious snacks:

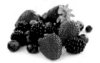 **Berries.** Berries are low in sugar and high in fiber. They are loaded with antioxidants, and have some anti-cancer properties (according to the American Cancer Society).

They are also tasty, and children love them! Serve out of the carton (preferably organic, and always washed).

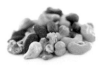 **Go Nuts!** Everyone likes a salty, crunchy snack. Instead of chips, choose nuts. They are high in protein and fiber, and when used in moderation, are associated with decreased heart disease. Serve by the (small) handful, or mix with GF cereal and a bit of dark chocolate for a nutritious bridge mix.

 An Apple a Day? Apples average 5 grams of fiber a piece, and have many nutrients, including bone-building vitamin K. They also have the anti-inflammatory nutrient, quercetin. They are filling and fun to crunch. Buy organic when possible, and always wash (but do not peel). Serve whole, or slice and serve with a dip. For a filling snack and some good protein, spread apple slices with a natural nut butter.

 Snacking "Eggs-"cellence" Keep some peeled, hard-boiled eggs in the fridge. Some consider eggs the perfect food, and they do make a great snack. High in protein and relatively low in calories, eggs also contain choline (important for heart and brain function) and Vitamin D, which many are deficient in. Add salt and pepper, and eggs are good to go!

 Pomegranates and Juice. This yummy juice is loaded with antioxidants, and can reduce blood pressure and plaque in the arteries. Serve with snacks or make a smoothie with this juice. You can buy the juice at any grocery store. The fruit is available seasonally, and is fun (though messy) to eat. Toss some of the pips into a salad for a surprising addition.

 Don't Assume ... your children will not eat vegetables! Keep cleaned vegetables ready to eat in the fridge. Most children will enjoy the crunch of carrot or cauliflower, especially if there is something good to dip it in. Try veggies with salsa or hummus (see recipe on page 279).

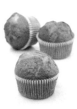 **Mini Muffins:** Easy to make, freeze, and eat. Children love small foods, so if your children are young, make mini muffins. Sneak in nutrition ... extra eggs or nuts for protein, flaxseed for omega fatty acids, and molasses and dried fruit for iron. Make a bunch and freeze for later. Muffin-top pans are great for some children. (Muffin tops are like soft cookies!)

Snack Mixes

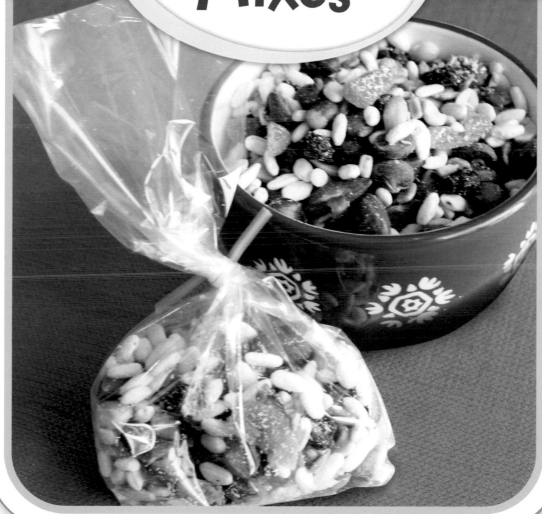

Gorp, recipe on page 145

Crunchy Mix

6 tablespoons olive oil

2 tablespoons GF
Worcestershire sauce
(see recipe in chapter 11)

1½ teaspoons kosher salt

¾ teaspoon garlic powder

½ teaspoon onion powder

3 cups Corn Crunch-Ems cereal

3 cups Rice Crunch-Ems cereal

1 cup GF pretzels

1 cup mixed nuts (optional)

It was such a boon to GF cereal lovers when Health Valley introduced their "Crunch-Ems" line of products. Although the rice version contains a minute amount of cornstarch, it is well tolerated even by individuals with corn sensitivities, and is worth a try. If needed, you can omit Corn Crunch-Ems. **Note:** Since first publishing this recipe, General Mills has removed gluten from their Chex line of cereal (with the exception of Wheat Chex and Multibran Chex), so feel free to use these cereals instead.

1 Preheat oven to 250°F.

2 Pour oil in a large roasting pan. Warm in oven for 5 minutes.

3 Stir seasonings into oil. Gradually stir in remaining ingredients until evenly coated.

4 Bake crunchy mix for 1 hour, stirring every 15 minutes.

5 Spread mix on paper towels to cool.

6 Store in airtight container.

Makes 16 servings

Gorp

I am not sure how trail mix came to be called *gorp*—some contend that it stands for Good Old Raisins and Peanuts. It is always a good idea to have gorp when you hit the trail, and sometimes I think it is the reason Sam likes to hike so much. Here is a recipe for gorp, but remember, anything you like is a good addition to gorp.

1 Mix all ingredients in a large bowl.
2 Store in serving-sized plastic bags until ready to eat.

Makes 16 servings

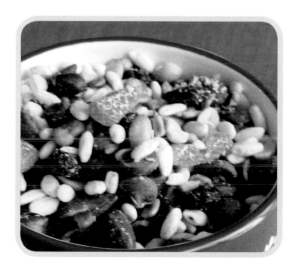

1 cup nuts, roasted and salted
1 cup raisins
1 cup puffed rice cereal
1 cup sunflower seeds
1 cup dried, shredded coconut (sulfite-free)
1 cup dried apricots, chopped
1 cup GFCF chocolate lentils* (or 1 cup GFCF chocolate chips)

M&M's contain milk and are forbidden, but it is possible to find the same type of candy in a dairy-free version. Check stores that have good supplies of kosher foods. Bloomy's is a brand that is widely available, but there are many others.

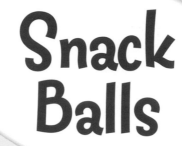

Snack Balls

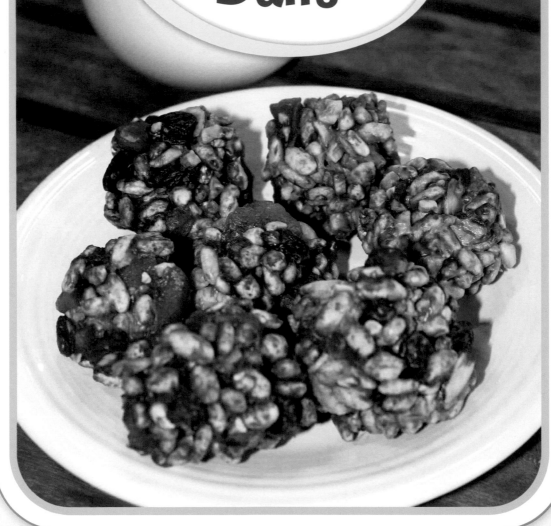

Cereal Munch Balls, recipe on page 147

Cereal Munch Balls

Here is a sweet treat that would be appropriate around Halloween when other children are eating sweet, goopy treats. Use any nut that is tolerated, or omit nuts if necessary.

3 cups puffed rice cereal
1 cup dried apricots, chopped
1 cup raisins
1 cup peanuts, dry-roasted
1 cup GFCF chocolate chips
⅓ cup CF margarine
1 cup nut butter (e.g., peanut, almond, cashew butter)

1 In a large bowl, combine cereal, apricots, raisins, peanuts, and chocolate chips.
2 In a microwave-safe 9"x13" baking dish, melt margarine on high for 2 minutes.
3 Stir margarine and add nut butter. Microwave on high 2 minutes longer. Stir until blended.
4 Add cereal mixture to nut butter mixture. Toss until well coated.
5 Working quickly with greased hands, form into balls, using about ½ cup cereal mixture per ball. If mixture begins to cool and harden, microwave on high 30 seconds or until softened.

Makes 36 servings

Variation: Omit peanut butter and margarine, toss ingredients together, and you have gorp!

Cowboy Bean Dip, recipe on page 159

✳ *new* Coconut Date Balls

1½ cups pitted dates
¾ cup coconut butter
   (or other nut butter)
1 tablespoon coconut oil
   (more if using nut butter)
1¼ cups finely shredded, dried
   coconut, divided

This is another recipe from Julie Matthews. Delicious and naturally sweet, these coconut balls pack a powerful nutritional punch. Be sure not to confuse the coconut butter with coconut oil — it is not the same thing. You can get coconut butter (or spread, as it is sometimes called) at most health food stores. This snack also has the benefit of being a "no-cook" recipe, which busy parents will appreciate!

1 In a food processor or high-end blender, process dates into a paste. Add coconut butter and coconut oil, and mix by pulsing. Next, add ¼ cup shredded coconut, and pulse further.
2 Roll mixture into balls. If balls are oily enough, shredded coconut should stick to outside of mixture.
3 Place remaining shredded coconut in a shallow bowl. Press balls into coconut. (If balls are drier, melt some coconut oil in a pan and roll balls in coconut oil, then roll in shredded coconut.)
4 Store in refrigerator.

Makes 6–8 servings

Lemon Power Balls

This recipe is very similar to Julie's, but the lemon flavor will be a real favorite for some. Try both and see which your family likes better. If desired, you can add 1–2 teaspoons of calcium powder to the mixture. The sesame seeds add calcium.

1 Process all ingredients (except coconut) in a blender or food processor.
2 Because this is a slightly sticky mixture, wet your hands first. Then, roll mixture into balls. If desired, roll balls in coconut.
3 Store in refrigerator.

Makes 6–8 servings

1 cup pitted dates, chopped
1 cup walnuts, chopped
¾ cup white sesame seeds
¼ cup fresh lemon juice
Grated zest from 2 lemons
½ cup unsweetened coconut
   flakes (optional)

Fruit Snacks

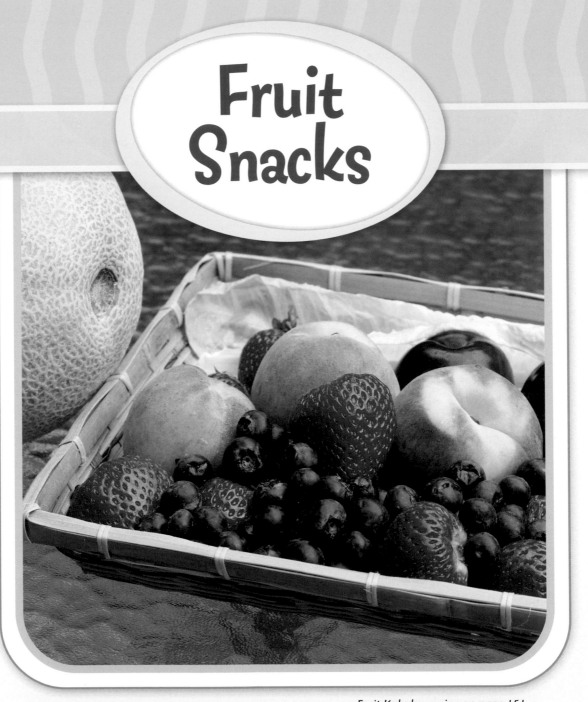

Fruit Kabobs, recipe on page 151

Fruit Kabobs

Most children like fresh fruit, and what could be more fun than fruit on a stick? If desired, roll the finished kabobs in coconut just before serving. Messy, but good! This is a fun thing to bring to a picnic. (If your children are young, beware of the pointy skewers.)

1 Clean all fruit, and cut into appropriate chunks.
2 Thread thin bamboo skewers with fruit chunks to make kabobs.
3 Sprinkle finished kabobs with a little lemon juice if not serving immediately.
4 Coat with coconut if desired.

Servings will vary.

Melon, cubed (or scooped
    with melon baller)
Pineapple chunks
Seedless grapes
Apple, cubed
Pear, cubed
Strawberries, hulled
Lemon juice
Shredded coconut (optional)

Stuffed Apples

1 apple
Peanut butter (or other
   nut butter)
Raisins
Sunflower seeds
Toasted coconut

Here is another odd recipe, but it is worth a try for the pickiest of young children. It has protein and fiber, too. If your child cannot tolerate apples, try using a very firm pear.

1 Preheat oven to 350°F.
2 Core apple, and stuff with nut butter.
3 Top with as much of remaining ingredients as you can. The filling will keep fruit from turning brown.
4 Bake for 30 minutes.

Makes 1 serving

Blueberry-Applesauce Fruit Leather

Fruit leather is a chewy, delicious dried-fruit treat. The sugars, acids, fiber, and nutrients found in fruit become concentrated when the water is removed. This makes dried fruits high in sugar, but the vitamins and mineral content is also high. Dried fruits provide a nutritious way to satisfy a sweet tooth.

Blueberries, pureed to make 1 cup
1 cup unsweetened applesauce
1 tablespoon honey

1 Preheat oven to 140°F if oven-drying fruit leather.
2 Combine all ingredients, and spread evenly on plastic wrap.
3 Dry fruit using a food dehydrator (follow manufacturer's instructions) or your oven. To oven-dry, use an oven thermometer to test temperature. Too high of a heat will melt plastic. Leave oven door ajar so moisture can escape. It takes about 6 hours to dry fruit leather in oven, but always test for dryness.
4 To make sure fruit leather is completely dried, try to pull leather from plastic wrap. If it peels from plastic and holds its shape, it is dry. (Insufficiently dried fruit will not keep well.)
5 When dry, roll fruit leather loosely in plastic wrap.
6 Place fruit leather in an airtight container. It will keep for more than 1 year if refrigerated or frozen.

Makes 4 servings

Frozen
Snacks

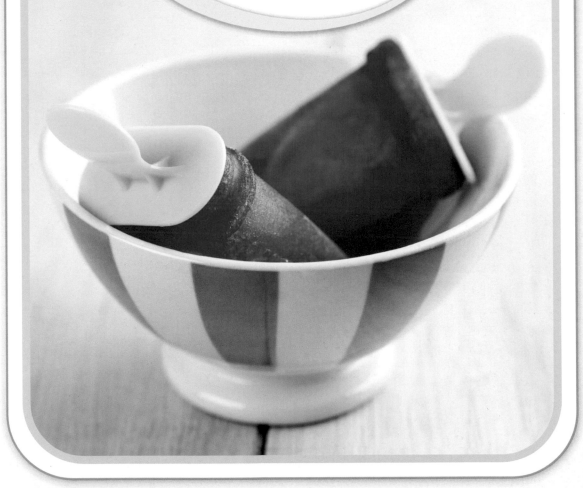

Frozen Fruit Pops, recipe on page 156

Frozen Banana Pops

I first experienced frozen bananas at Dairy Queen when I was very young. I hear they still have these treats! They are easy enough to make, and fun to eat. If your child tolerates bananas, they make a great summertime treat. I always use DariFree™ for this recipe, but any milk substitute should do. I think coconut milk might work especially well.

2 bananas
1 cup GFCF chocolate chips
2 tablespoons milk substitute
1 tablespoon solid shortening
   (e.g., Spectrum brand)

1 Peel bananas, and cut them in half.

2 Insert a skewer (or stick) into each banana.

3 In double boiler or microwave, melt chocolate chips with milk substitute and shortening.

4 Dip banana chunks into chocolate and cool on wax paper.

5 When banana pops are hardened, wrap well and freeze.

Makes 4 servings

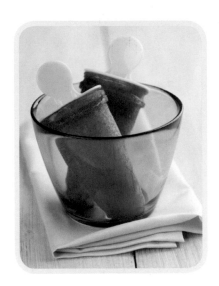

 # Frozen Fruit Pops

Most children love fruit, but it is even better when it is frozen into a pop! Unfortunately, most fruit pops, even the ones labeled "no added sugar," contain something you are trying to avoid. They cost a fortune, too. It is cheap and easy to make your own, and you can use fruit (or combination of fruits) your family likes best. You can probably even slip in a veggie or two without anyone being the wiser. If you do not have any plastic pop molds (available everywhere), paper cups and wooden craft sticks will work fine. Frozen pops are a delicious, wholesome snack, especially good in summer when wonderful fruit is available.

2 cups fruit, chopped
1 tablespoon sugar
   (or sweetener of your
   choice)
1 teaspoon lemon juice
   (or lime juice)
Piece of carrot or other
   vegetable (optional)
Water (optional)

1 Put all ingredients in a blender or food processor, and blend until smooth. (To make pops slushier before freezing, add 1 tablespoon water to mixture.)
2 Pour mixture into 4 pop molds, and freeze.

Makes 4 servings

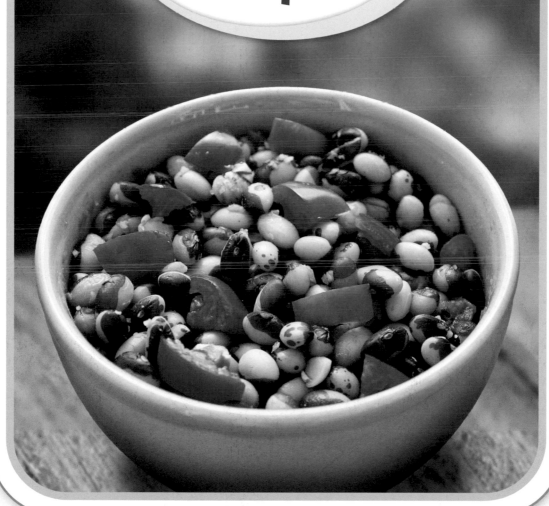

Snack Dips

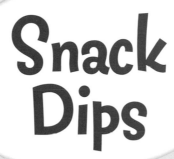

Cowboy Bean Dip, recipe on page 159

✳ new Bean Dip

1 (16-ounce) can beans
   (I like black beans, but use
   whatever you like)
1 (7-ounce) bottle roasted red
   pepper (or from store's
   salad bar)
1 garlic clove, finely minced
2 tablespoons olive oil
2 teaspoons balsamic vinegar
Salt and pepper (to taste)

This is a very easy dip to put together, and delicious with chips — or better yet, vegetable sticks. I serve this in its natural (chunky) state, but you could purée the dip in a blender if you prefer a smooth texture.

1 Mix all ingredients together.
2 Chill or serve at room temperature.

Makes 6–8 servings

Cowboy Bean Dip

I have no idea why this is called "Cowboy Bean Dip," but perhaps it is because cowboys often ride Pinto horses. This dip can be made with canned beans, of course, but if you plan ahead, you could cook your own beans. It is easy, you just have to remember to soak them ahead of time. My two favorite sources for an incredibly wide variety of beans are Ranchogordo.com and Purcellmountainfarms.com. Some of these beans are so beautiful, you will not want to purée them all (but if your children will not eat chunky foods, you will have to!).

1 (15-ounce) can pinto beans, divided
1 cup salsa (mild or medium)
½ cup onion, chopped
2 teaspoons lemon juice

1 Combine all ingredients (except ½ cup beans), and purée in blender or food processor.
2 Add reserved beans to give dip some chunks if desired. (If not, purée all beans.)
3 Chill or serve dip at room temperature.

Servings will vary.

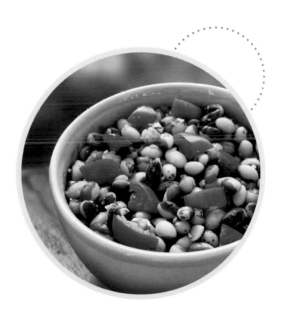

Other Snacktime Favorites

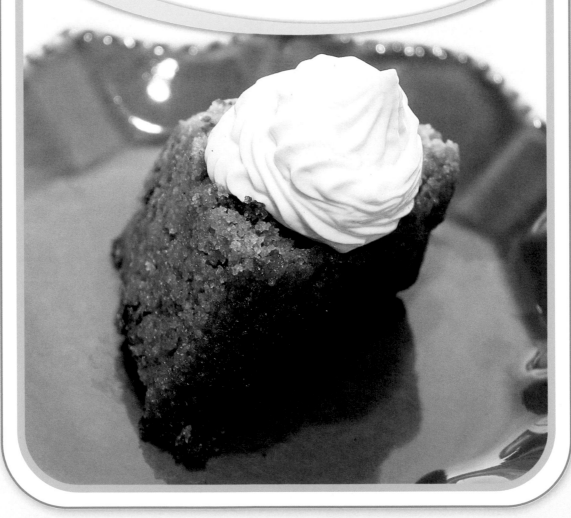

Raisin Snack Cake, recipe on page 161
Topped with Cashew Cream, recipe on page 348

Raisin Snack Cake

Ever since I read Louise Fitzhugh's *Harriet the Spy* when I was in fifth grade, I have loved the idea of cake and milk after school. This cake is very simple, and just sweet enough to be good. It is a great afterschool snack with a big glass of DariFree™. It makes a good lunchbox addition, too. I love to use dried fruits other than raisins when I bake; I usually have dried cherries, cranberries, and blueberries on hand.

1 Preheat oven to 350°F.

2 Bring water to a boil, and add raisins.

3 Remove from heat, and let raisins "steep" for about 10 minutes, then cool.

4 Combine remaining ingredients with raisins, and mix well.

5 Bake cake in 10″ square pan for 30–35 minutes, or until it tests done. (If you use a loaf pan, bake cake for 50–55 minutes.)

Makes 6–8 servings

2 cups water

1 cup raisins (or other dried fruit)

1 cup GF flour blend

¾ cup sorghum flour

½ cup CF margarine

½ cup sugar

½ cup nuts, chopped

2 teaspoons xanthan gum

1 teaspoon pure vanilla extract

1 teaspoon GF baking soda

1 teaspoon cinnamon

½ teaspoon nutmeg (preferably freshly grated)

½ teaspoon salt

Kiddie Kibbles

1 recipe GF garlic croutons
   (see recipe on page 328)
½ cup olive oil
2 teaspoons sesame seeds
1 teaspoon celery seeds
1 teaspoon salt
1 teaspoon imported sweet
   paprika

Everyone knows that the croutons are the best part of a salad. So why not just cut to the chase and snack on the croutons? I call these snacks kibbles because they remind me of my dog's crunchy food.

1 Preheat oven to 275°F.

2 Pour croutons into large bowl. Combine remaining ingredients in a separate bowl, and toss with croutons.

3 Place croutons on baking sheet.

4 Toast croutons for 20 minutes, stirring every 5 minutes.

5 Allow to cool, and serve.

Servings will vary.

Ants on a Log

Your children have probably made these at school—nearly everyone does. They are fun to make and eat. Feel free to use a different nut butter, or if nut is not tolerated, you can use tahini (sesame paste).

Celery stalk
Peanut butter
Raisins

1 Fill center of celery with peanut butter.
2 Place raisins on top and serve.

Makes 1 serving

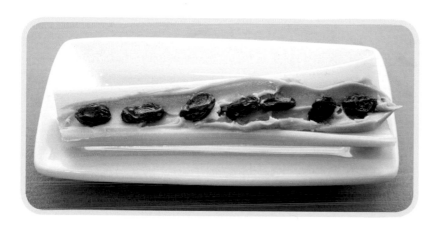

Nut Bars

1½ cups sorghum flour

¾ cup brown sugar, packed

½ cup CF margarine, melted
  (or coconut butter)

2 teaspoons xanthan gum

1 cup GFCF chocolate chips

½ cup pure cane syrup
  (or rice syrup)

3 tablespoons ghee

1 (12-ounce) can salted nuts
  (about 2 cups)

These delicious nut bars are packed with protein. If nuts are tolerated, they make a terrific snack. They lend themselves to flour substitution, so if you rotate grains, do not feel that sorghum is your only choice. Use whatever nuts your family likes and tolerates. A mixture of more than one kind of nut works well. If using coconut butter in place of CF margarine, be sure not to confuse it with coconut oil — it is not the same thing. You can get coconut butter (or spread, as it is sometimes called) at most health food stores.

1 Preheat oven to 350°F.

2 In a medium bowl, combine flour, sugar, margarine, and xanthan gum (mixture will be crumbly).

3 Press mixture into an ungreased 13"x9"x2" baking pan.

4 Bake crust for 12 minutes.

5 Sprinkle nuts over baked crust.

6 In a small saucepan, heat chocolate chips, cane syrup, and ghee over low heat, stirring to prevent burning.

7 When melted, drizzle chocolate mixture evenly over crust, then add nuts on top.

8 Return bars to oven and bake for 8 minutes more.

9 Cut bars while warm and serve.

Makes 12 bars

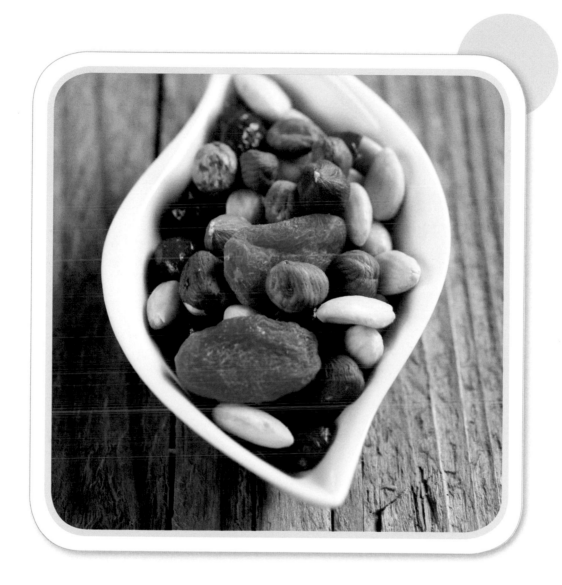

CHAPTER 8

Dinnertime: Main Dishes and Sides

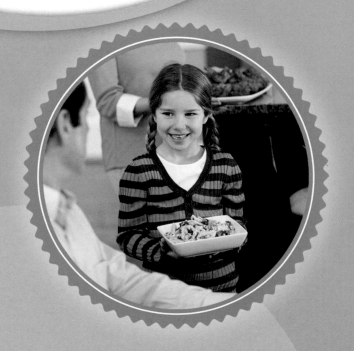

I have been cooking family dinners for a long time, and for me, the hardest part of making dinner is thinking of something to make. I am not the kind of person who makes six or seven meals that get cycled through the week, and my family is easily bored with repeats! For me, the Internet was the best thing that ever happened to dinner because I can enter a few search terms and come up with a fresh idea or new technique.

When I was newer to cooking, however, I did rely on books (and long distance calls to my mom). Most parents today find it hard to find the time to make a home-cooked, nutritious dinner. Between school meetings, sports events, and extra-curricular activities, making and sitting down to a family meal may well be headed for extinction. When you add to that a child with special needs, you have to also factor in therapy sessions, doctor's appointments, and parental exhaustion. Having some "go-to" family meals at your fingertips should help a lot, and that is what this chapter provides.

In this chapter I have tried to come up with many ideas for dinner, but beyond that I have tried to emphasize main dishes that are simple to put together. My goal is to present super-easy recipes that look (and taste) as if they took much more effort than you actually expended. I hope that some of the recipes in this chapter will prove to be family favorites. Whenever possible, they should provide more than one meal (either as leftovers or transformed into a casserole or soup).

For some of these "easy" dishes (often named "The World's Easiest...."), I use prepared foods like salsa or canned beans. If you try a recipe that calls for such an ingredient, always read the label carefully to be sure that you are buying food without a lot of artificial ingredients or additives. I also have included many dishes that are inherently simple. Roasting a chicken is scary at first, but once you have done it once or twice, it will be a favorite meal. If you have a barbeque, you can prepare foods without a lot of fancy sauces or breading, and it will always taste great. (We grill year-round, dashing outside to turn food during cold weather!)

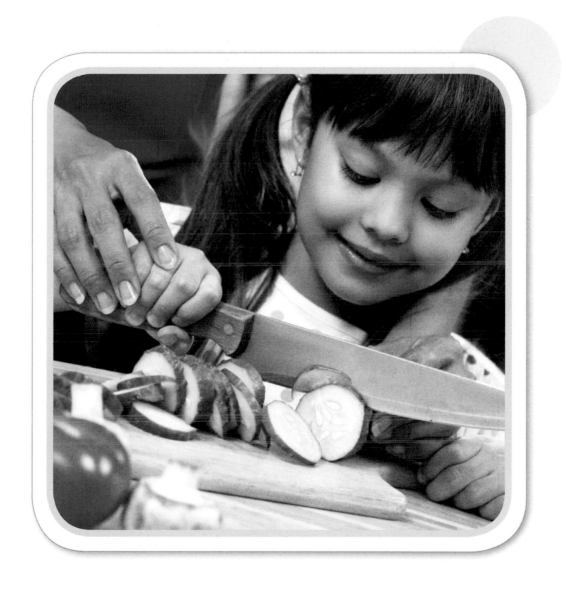

Mains

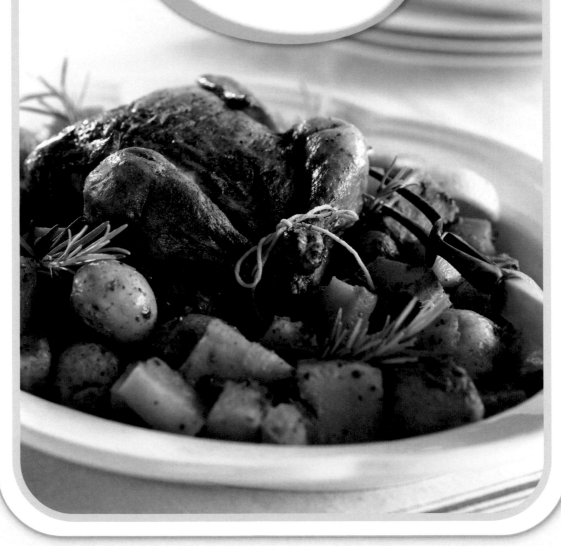

Roast Chicken, recipe on page 172

Chicken "Nuggets"

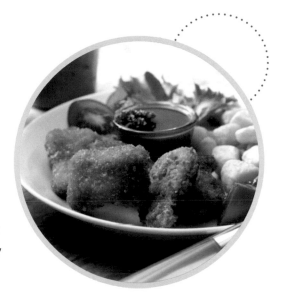

No, they are not from you-know-where, but they are delicious. Your children should love them — these nuggets never last long around our house. Since you can make as many or as few as you want, I give no measurements for this recipe. But my advice is — make a lot! They freeze and reheat beautifully. If your child is off grains, "bread" the nuggets in coarsely ground nut meal. If your children are not already addicted to breaded chicken (or even if they are!), try to teach them to eat plain, grilled chicken strips. Sometimes this is more acceptable if you offer a dipping sauce. Even if you are not currently limiting starches and grains, this is a good direction in which to take your children's diets.

1 Slice chicken into strips, then into bite-sized chunks.
2 Beat egg lightly with water, and pour into a shallow pan or pie plate.
3 In another shallow dish, season bread crumb mix with spices.
4 Dip chicken pieces first into egg, and then coat well in crumb mixture. Roll each dipped piece in the breading, and coat well.
5 Fry chicken in very hot oil, about ½" deep, until golden brown on all sides. Drain well on paper towel-lined plates.
6 Serve while warm. Extras that have been frozen reheat well.

Servings will vary.

Fish Sticks Variation: Cut any firm-fleshed, white fish into "sticks" and treat as you would boneless, skinless chicken breast meat.

Boneless, skinless chicken breast
1 egg (or melted CF margarine or milk substitute)
2 tablespoons water
GF bread crumb mix*
Salt, pepper, garlic powder, and onion powder (optional)
Canola oil (or coconut oil)

 *There are many excellent GF bread crumb mixes available now (check resource list on page 356). If you prefer, blend your favorite GF crispy rice cracker or cereal with some sulfite-free mashed potato flakes (e.g., Barbara's brand), salt, pepper, and any spices you like.

✻ₙₑw Roast Chicken

1 (5–6-pound) roasting chicken

2 tablespoons olive oil, divided

Sea salt

Freshly ground pepper

1 lemon, cut into quarters
   (or orange)

Sprig of thyme (optional)

4 large garlic cloves, peeled but
   left whole

1 large yellow onion, sliced

4 carrots, peeled and cut into
   2" chunks (or small package
   baby carrots)

3 white potatoes, peeled and
   sliced thickly (optional)

Everyone should know how to roast a chicken. It is easy and delicious, and you can use the leftover meat in casseroles, stews, and soups. The carcass can be boiled to make homemade broth. If you can afford to, buy organic chicken. If you cannot (and they are more expensive), try to buy chicken that has not been injected or doctored in any way with chemicals, preservatives, or colorings. A basic roast chicken makes a great Sunday (or any day) dinner, and is good enough to prepare for company or holidays. There are many ways to make a roasted chicken; the following technique works every time. Should you buy a chicken with one of those pop-up thermometers, remember the lesson I learned from my brother-in-law: When the thermometer pops, it tells you that the chicken is overdone!

1 Preheat oven to 425°F.

2 Remove bag of giblets from inside of chicken and set aside for your cat, or to make gravy.

3 Wash chicken, inside and out. Pat dry and remove any excess fat.

4 Brush chicken with 1 tablespoon olive oil, then salt and pepper inside and out.

5 Stuff fruit, herbs, and garlic into chicken and tie legs together with string or kitchen "rubber bands," which are available in kitchen stores (unwaxed dental floss works in a pinch).

6 Put onion, carrots, and potatoes in the bottom of a roasting pan large enough to accommodate your bird, and add salt, pepper and 1 tablespoon olive oil on vegetables.

7 Toss vegetables to coat, then place bird on top, breast-side up.

8 Roast chicken for about 90 minutes. The internal temperature should be 160°F, and juices should run clear when pierced with a knife between leg and thigh. A larger chicken will take longer to roast, so be sure to check the internal temperature.

9 Check chicken after 1 hour. If it is getting too brown, cover lightly with foil.

10 When done, cover with foil and let chicken rest for 15 minutes. This allows juices to come back into meat, and is an important step.

11 Carve as you would a turkey. (Check Youtube.com if you need a guide.)

Servings will vary.

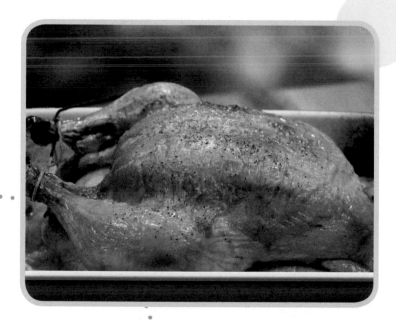

Roasted Cornish Hens

4 (1-pound) Cornish hens

4 garlic cloves, peeled and
   crushed

¼ cup olive oil

1 tablespoon sea salt

1 teaspoon dried thyme

1 teaspoon dried rosemary

1 teaspoon coarsely ground
   black pepper

20 fingerling or small new
   potatoes (optional)

Cornish hens are just little chickens. Older children and adults can generally eat a whole bird; small children can be expected to eat ¼ – ½ of a hen. This recipe makes 4 hens, but if you need more or fewer, adjust accordingly. I always buy the smallest hens I can find.

1 Preheat oven to 375°F.

2 Rinse hens and pat dry, then place in a roasting pan.

3 Carefully loosen skin from birds, and spoon garlic directly on flesh of breast. (Be careful not to tear skin, and remove any sharp rings before attempting.)

4 Brush birds with olive oil and then season with salt, herbs, and pepper.

5 Roast for 40 minutes, then place potatoes around birds and return to oven for another 45–50 minutes. When done, skin should be crispy and brown.

Makes 4–6 servings

Moist Chicken Breasts

Sometimes you want to make Chicken and Dumplings or another recipe that calls for cooked chicken meat, but you do not have any leftovers. No problem—this is an easy way to make chicken for other uses. Though it is healthier not to eat the delicious, crispy skin, the chicken will be moister if you cook it with the skin on. Just remove the skin when you are done cooking.

Chicken breasts, bone in
Olive oil
Sea salt
Freshly ground pepper

1 Preheat the oven to 350°F.

2 Line a sheet pan with foil to make clean-up easier, and place chicken breasts on pan.

3 Brush with olive oil, then season with salt and pepper.

4 Roast for 40 minutes, or until the meat is cooked through.

5 If you are using chicken for another recipe, let cool enough to handle. Remove skin and chop meat as directed for your recipe.

Servings will vary.

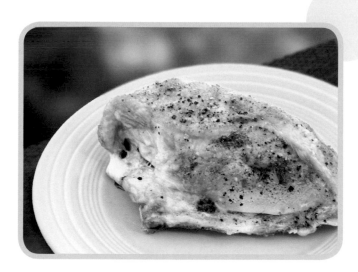

How to Butterfly a Bird

This is really just a variation on our chicken theme, but it is a terrific technique to know, especially if your time is limited. A bird is said to be *butterflied* when its' backbone (and sometimes breast bone) is removed, and the bird is flattened. Because this flattening greatly increases the surface area of the bird relative to its volume, it will cook very quickly.

For a small bird, it can take as little as 20 minutes to cook, and even a large turkey can be roasted in under 1 hour. This technique is great for grilling too — a regular fryer can be butterflied and then cooked outside. To save time, you can butterfly and marinate a bird the night before. When you come home, heat up the grill and voila — a crispy, delicious dish that will earn you instant induction into the dinnertime hall of fame!

There are just a few steps to butterflying a bird, and they are the same no matter the size of the bird. To see it done, search Youtube.com.

You will need sharp kitchen shears or a good boning knife.

Steps

1 Place the bird, breast-side down, with the legs pointing toward you.

2 Use your fingers to feel for the backbone. Then, use the scissors to cut down one side of the backbone, staying as close to the outside of the backbone as you can. You can hold on to the tail of the chicken while cutting to keep the bird from sliding on the cutting surface.

3 When you reach the neck, do the same thing on the other side of the backbone.

4 The backbone can now be easily removed.

5 You can spread the ribs apart and continue, but many people choose to remove the breast bone (or keel) as well. If you remove the keel, you will be able to flatten out the bird without so much "bone crunching," and it will be easy to divide in half for serving.

6 To remove the breastbone, turn the chicken so that the legs are now pointing away from you, and look for the white spot at the top of the bird. This is the top of the bone you want to remove.

7 Make a cut in this spot, and then you will be able to bend back both sides of the bird to expose the breastbone.

8 When the breastbone is exposed, you can easily remove it, usually just with your hands. You should be able to "pop" it out with your fingers after you have loosened it from the meat.

9 Use a paring knife or your shears to remove any excess fat or tissue, then wash the bird and pat dry before seasoning and cooking.

10 Be sure to tuck the wings under the breast to keep them from burning.

I find that for small birds, it is nicer to remove the breastbone, but for a very large bird, such as a turkey, I leave the keel in. For a turkey, which will take about 45 minutes to roast, you want to put the wings over the breast (to keep them from drying), and spread the legs apart.

Remember, chickens and turkeys should have an internal temperature of 155°F–165°F. An instant-read thermometer is an excellent gadget to have in the kitchen. Butterflied birds should be rubbed with olive oil and seasoned just like whole birds. ★

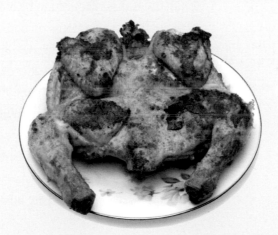

✹ Roast Turkey

Equipment

18"x 20" roasting pan, 2" deep (disposable pans are not strong enough)
Adjustable rack that fits the pan
Instant-read thermometer
Clean dish towel

Ingredients

Fresh turkey (not frozen)
Water
Salt and pepper (to taste)

 The Butterball Turkey Hotline maintains that their most common question concerns cooking the turkey with the bag of giblets still inside the bird!

The fastest way to roast a turkey is by using the "butterfly" technique (see page 176). Last year my Thanksgiving turkey took just under 1 hour to cook. For some people, this method just will not work for Thanksgiving or Christmas because the bird is not whole and available for oohing and aahing and at-table carving demonstrations. So how do you roast a turkey in a more traditional manner? There are many ways to do it, and everyone has their favorite method (my brother-in-law roasts his bird in a paper bag every Thanksgiving and, yes, sometimes they catch fire!) Google "how to roast a turkey" and you will find hundreds of articles on the subject. Personally, though, I prefer the Fast Roast method. If I have pies, dressing, potatoes, and other holiday dishes that need to be baked, I do not want to tie up the oven for hours on end roasting a bird. Using this method, a turkey will cook in about 8 minutes per pound; a 14-pound bird will cook in 90 minutes. Be sure that your oven is very clean, or you will set off every smoke alarm in the neighborhood!

1 Set oven rack to its lowest level. Preheat oven to 500°F 30 minutes before you are ready to roast turkey.
2 Place rack in roasting pan, adjusted to its lowest position.
3 Remove giblets* from inside turkey and rinse bird, inside and out.
4 Place turkey breast-side up on the rack and cover with a clean towel. **Leave at room temperature for at least 2 hours.**
5 Remove the towel. Do not stuff the bird ("stuffing" can be baked later in a casserole). Do not truss, skewer,

or tie up bird; instead, you want to spread legs apart (taking care not to break the skin).

6 Place pan in oven with legs facing oven door. Let cook for 45 minutes. Do not open oven door during this time. After 45 minutes, if there is smoke coming from oven, pour 1 cup lukewarm water into the pan. Do not baste bird, but do open windows and doors if necessary, and use your oven's exhaust fan.

7 When bird is brown, cover loosely with foil. After 1 hour, check the internal temperature with thermometer by sticking it into the thickest part of the thigh (do not touch the bone). The turkey should be removed from the oven when the internal temperature is between 165–170°F.

8 Remove bird and let rest for 20 minutes before carving. Resting is very important! The bird will continue to cook and the internal temperature will rise between 5 and 10 degrees. Resting also lets juices come back into meat so you do not lose all the moisture to the cutting board.

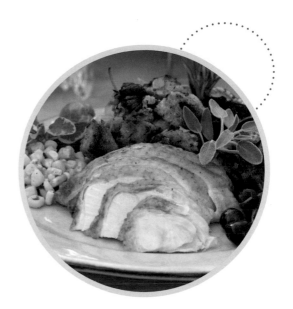

Servings will vary.

Note: If you want to make gravy, cook giblets and neck in a saucepan with 6 cups chicken stock. If it simmers until it reduces to 4 cups (this takes at least 1 hour), you should not need to add any thickener.

The turkey was not seasoned before roasting, so do add some salt and pepper to bird when it comes out of oven.

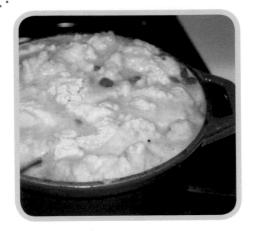

World's Easiest Chicken and Dumplings

Chicken and dumplings may be one of the greatest "comfort foods" I know of, but it does not have to be a big deal to make. This recipe will work well with leftover chicken (e.g., from roast chicken). In the first publication of this recipe, I listed soy cheese as an optional ingredient, but none of the soy cheeses were actually very good, and many children cannot tolerate soy. I had pretty much given up recommending anything that needed a cheese substitute until Daiya came along. This is a fantastic CF vegan cheese substitute that tastes good and actually melts like cheese. It can be used in any recipe, and you can find it at Whole Foods and other specialty markets. Visit their website (see resource list on page 356) to find a store near you that carries this fantastic new ingredient! You can easily omit the cheese and still have a delicious dish.

1 (32-ounce) container
   Imagine Cream of Potato
   and Leek Soup
1 (16-ounce) package mixed
   frozen vegetables
   (your choice)
½–1 cup Daiya "cheese"
   (optional)
4 large pieces or 6 small pieces
   cooked chicken
   (e.g., 4 breasts)
1 teaspoon arrowroot starch
   (optional)

Chicken

1 Heat the soup to a boil in a 4-quart saucepan. Add vegetables and cook over medium heat until it returns to a boil.

2 Lower to a simmer and cook for about 10 minutes. (The exact cooking time will depend on your choice of vegetables and their size).

3 Add Daiya cheese and cook until melted.

4 Cut chicken into bite-size pieces, add to the pot, and heat through.

5 If you want a thicker stew, or if you do not add the optional cheese, remove about 4 ounces liquid from saucepan, and stir arrowroot starch into it. Be sure that all lumps are dissolved, then add mixture back to pot.

Makes 4 servings

Dumplings

1 Combine flour mix, baking powder, and salt in a medium bowl.

2 Using a pastry blender or two knives, cut in shortening until mixture resembles coarse cornmeal.

3 Slowly add milk substitute and mix until you have a soft, thick dough.

4 With a large spoon or wet hands, form dumplings and place on top of gently boiling chicken mixture.

5 Cook for 10 minutes uncovered, then cover the pot and cook for an additional 10 minutes.

Makes 4 servings

Variation: Don't like (or have time to make) dumplings? Serve this over rice or GF noodles instead.

1 cup Gifts of Nature GF flour mix*

1½ teaspoon GF baking powder

Salt (to taste)

2 tablespoons shortening

½ cup milk substitute

You can use other GF flour mixes, but this one works particularly well.

Simple Chicken Stew

Chicken
Oil
GF chicken or vegetable broth
Sweet rice flour (available at
    Chinese groceries)
Vegetables (your choice)
GFCF miso paste

 Note: *Miso is a fermented food, so check with your doctor if you are not sure whether or not to use it; many children on yeast-free diets must avoid fermented foods. Read the ingredients carefully, as some pastes are made with barley. These pastes are high in protein and extremely flavorful. There are even rice misos available, although they are harder to find. A small dollop greatly improves the flavor of a large pot of soup or stew. Miso paste can be found in the refrigerator section of most health food stores.*

This stew works well with boned, skinned breast meat (see Moist Chicken Breasts recipe on page 175) and is another good comfort food. Actually, it is not exactly a recipe because no specific amounts are given. Determine the ingredients you use, based on what your family likes. Quantities needed are based on the amount of meat you are cooking. It is OK to "wing it" when cooking!

1 In a heavy skillet at least 3″ deep, brown chicken in 1 tablespoon oil. If the meat sticks, add some GF chicken stock. While the meat is browning, sprinkle in a few teaspoons of sweet rice flour.

2 When the meat is browned, add broth to cover about ⅓ of meat. Add a few chopped onions, potatoes, carrots, or any other vegetable your family likes. Then add a few spoonfuls of miso paste. It is very salty, so take care not to add too much. If any lumps form, press them out with the back of a spoon.

3 Bring to a boil, then lower heat and cover.

4 Simmer the dish for 1 hour or until meat is cooked through and vegetables are tender. If the sauce is not thick enough, simmer uncovered.

5 Add peas, broccoli, or other quick-cooking vegetables during the last 10 minutes of cooking.

6 If boned meat is used, cut into bite-sized chunks when tender.

Servings will vary.

Pineapple Chicken

Pineapple is well tolerated by many children who are allergic to citrus fruits, and it often makes a nice alternative. Even when following a yeast-free regimen, pineapple is acceptable (in moderation). Likewise, coconut milk is a food to which few children react. If your family is limiting grains, the rice may be omitted, though it may not be as thick. This dish is mild and creamy.

1 Sauté onion in oil and cook until slightly brown.
2 Add spices and rice to pan and cook, stirring constantly, for about 2 minutes.
3 Add chicken and cook until brown.
4 Add broth and stir to mix.
5 Bring mixture to a simmer, then cover and cook over low heat for 20-30 minutes (until rice absorbs liquid).
6 Drain pineapple well, reserving juice. Stir arrowroot into juice in a small bowl to make a paste. Add coconut milk and pineapple chunks to the chicken, and then add the paste. The sauce will thicken almost immediately, but you will want to continue cooking and stirring over low heat until it gets very thick.

Makes 4 servings

1 teaspoon oil
1 onion, chopped
1 pound boneless chicken breast, cut into bite-sized chunks
¼ teaspoon ground ginger
Salt and pepper (to taste)
¼ cup uncooked rice
1 cup GF chicken broth
½ cup canned, unsweetened pineapple chunks, in juice
½ teaspoon arrowroot starch
1 (12-ounce) can light coconut milk

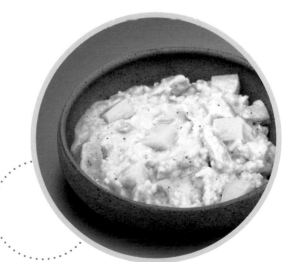

Brunswick Stew

1 chicken, cut into serving
    pieces
Cold water
1 onion, chopped
2 celery stalks, chopped
1 teaspoon dried marjoram
1 teaspoon dried oregano
2 cups frozen corn
    (substitute another
    vegetable if sensitive
    to corn)
1 cup canned butter beans,
    drained and rinsed
    (puree if your child will not
    eat beans)
1 (1-pound) box tomatoes
2 baking potatoes, peeled and
    cubed
2 tablespoons apple cider
    vinegar
1 tablespoon firmly packed
    brown sugar (optional)
⅓ cup GF ketchup
2 tablespoons CF margarine
½ teaspoon Tabasco sauce
Salt and pepper (to taste)

When I first started cooking, I was armed with only the 1967 edition of *The Joy of Cooking*. Brunswick Stew was one of the first things I cooked, though I am not really sure why. There are lots of variations on this traditional stew, but the one that follows is very good and can be made on the stove top or in a slow cooker.

1 Place chicken in a Dutch oven and add enough water to cover. Bring to a boil, removing any foam that forms. Add onion, celery, and spices, and boil until chicken is well cooked and nearly coming off the bones.

2 Remove chicken to a platter to cool.

3 Add remaining ingredients to broth and cook for about 1 hour (potatoes should be fork tender).

4 Remove chicken from bones and add it back to stew.

5 Let chicken heat through and serve.

Makes 4 servings

Curried Chicken Balls

Do not let the name fool you — this has just enough spice to be interesting. These make a nice change of pace from the usual chicken nugget — use strips for "tenders" if you prefer. Great for lunch or dinner. (These can also be fried.)

1 Preheat oven to 375°F.

2 Combine eggs and water in shallow bowl or pan. Beat to combine.

3 In a separate shallow pan (a pie plate works well), combine cereal and spices.

4 Dip pieces of chicken in egg, then coat with cereal mixture.

5 Place coated pieces on a foil-covered cookie sheet and spray lightly with cooking spray.

6 Bake for about 15 minutes or until chicken is tender and not pink.

Makes 4 servings

2 eggs
2 tablespoons water
3 cups GF crispy rice cereal,
    crushed to 1½ cups
    (use ground nuts for SCD)
1 teaspoon dried minced onion
½ teaspoon curry powder*
½ teaspoon garlic powder
Salt and pepper (to taste)
1 pound boneless chicken
    breast, cut into bite-sized
    pieces

 *If SCD or other carbohydrate reduced diet is being followed, spice blends like curry powder are generally avoided. You can add cumin, turmeric, and pepper (main ingredients in curry powder) separately.

Hungarian Chicken

1 chicken, cut into serving
  pieces
1 onion, diced
1 tablespoon olive oil
  (or CF margarine)
1 (15-ounce) container stewed
  tomatoes
2 tablespoons imported sweet
  paprika
1 teaspoon chili powder
1 garlic clove (or 1 teaspoon
  garlic powder)
2 tablespoons chili sauce
½ teaspoon dried basil
½ teaspoon dried parsley

This recipe is not, I fear, authentic Hungarian. It is good, however, and is quite easy to prepare. You can make this up to the point of baking, and store overnight.

1 Preheat oven to 375°F.
2 Brown chicken on a baking sheet for about 40 minutes. Lower oven temperature to 350°F.
3 In a saucepan, sauté onion in oil. When onions are soft, add remaining ingredients and cook for a few minutes over medium heat.
4 Place chicken in an ovenproof casserole, and cover with sauce. Then bake for 45–60 minutes.

Makes 4–6 servings

Buffalo Wings

My children love wings. They are easy to make, either baked in the oven or on the grill. The important thing is the marinade. Be sure to let wings marinate overnight if possible. The spiciness can be adjusted to your taste. Though traditionally served with blue cheese dressing, try the Ranch dressing recipe on page 330. Most recipes call for frying, but I like to grill or bake wings.

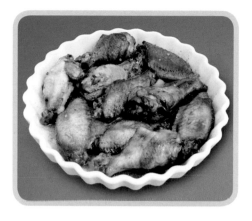

1 Preheat oven to 400°F.

2 Place all ingredients in a casserole dish or a large, strong plastic bag (a bag has the advantage that you can mix wings around every few hours without having to unwrap them) to marinate. If using a dish, be sure to cover tightly but unwrap and stir the wings around.

3 Refrigerate wings in marinade overnight.

4 Bake wings for 30–40 minutes or until done, or grill.

5 If grilling, use marinade to brush wings as they cook. If baking, add marinade as needed to prevent burning and sticking.

Makes 4–6 servings

4 pounds chicken wings

1 cup apple cider vinegar

2 tablespoons oil

2 tablespoons GF
   Worcestershire sauce*

1 teaspoon garlic powder

1 teaspoon chili powder

1 teaspoon salt

2–4 teaspoons Tabasco sauce
   (to taste)

 As of this writing, Lea & Perrins Worcestershire is GF. It does contain high fructose corn syrup, however, and other corn products. You may prefer to make your own Worcestershire sauce — see page 334 for recipe.

Arroz con Pollo

3 tablespoons olive oil

1 pound chicken
   (I prefer to use boned,
   skinless breast meat)

1 red bell pepper, chopped
   finely

1½ cups uncooked rice

3 cups chicken stock
   (homemade or GF canned)

1½ cups Pomi packaged
   tomatoes, with juice

1 tablespoon parsley, minced
   or dried

2 teaspoons paprika

1 teaspoon garlic, freshly
   minced (or use powder
   or bottled)

My friend Harriet Barnett has been GFCF cooking for her son Andrew for many years. I "met" her several years ago when I read a letter she had written to Bernard Rimland's ARI newsletter, looking for others following this regimen. I wrote to her and soon we were phone pals, speaking periodically. Later we switched to email and more regular communication; when her daughter was attending Princeton University, we managed to get together several times. She has shared many recipes with me over the years, and here is one of Andrew's favorites.

1 Heat olive oil and sauté chicken. Add pepper and rice, stirring to coat.

2 Add remaining ingredients and stir.

3 Bring to a boil, then lower heat, cover, and simmer for 25–30 minutes.

Makes 4–6 servings

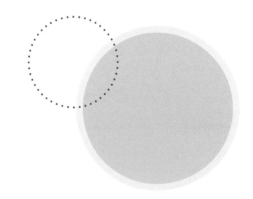

World's Easiest Chicken Curry

Not long ago, I roasted a 7-pound chicken on the grill. It was delicious, but there were only three of us at the table, so there were a lot of leftovers! The next night I tossed this simple curried dish together, made some rice, and the whole thing was done in 20 minutes. Curry does not have to be hot — my son prefers mild foods, so I went easy on the chilies. Adjust to your family's taste.

1 Sauté onion in 1 tablespoon oil.

2 When onion is soft but not browned, add garlic and ginger and cook over low heat for 2–3 minutes more. Stir often, as garlic tends to burn.

3 Add tomato paste, seasonings, and coconut milk. Cook over low heat until mixture starts to thicken, then add chicken.

4 Cook until sauce is quite thick and chicken is heated through.

5 Sprinkle with cilantro, and serve over rice.

Makes 4–6 servings

1 onion, sliced

2 tablespoons oil

2 garlic cloves, minced*

Small ginger knob, peeled and grated*

2 tablespoons tomato paste (from a tube)

1–3 teaspoons curry powder, according to taste

Salt, pepper, chilies (to taste)

1 (15-ounce) can coconut milk, regular or light

Cooked chicken meat, cubed with skin removed

Fresh cilantro* (optional)

 *Some stores carry Dorot brand frozen cubes of garlic, ginger, cilantro, and other herbs. I love the convenience of these cubes, and often use them in recipes like this. They preserve the flavor of the herbs, and are easy to toss into casseroles and other dishes. You can find them at Trader Joe's and some grocery stores.

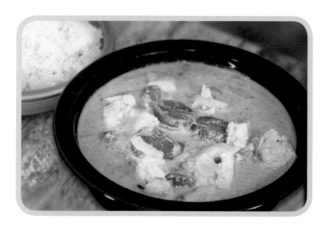

Baked Kibbe

1 pound ground lamb
3 tablespoons GF breadcrumbs
  (or cooked rice)
1 tablespoon onion, minced
1 teaspoon minced parsley
½ teaspoon salt
½ teaspoon ginger
½ teaspoon ground allspice
¼ teaspoon cumin
1 egg
2 garlic cloves, crushed
1 tablespoon pine nuts,
  toasted

Kibbe is a Middle-Eastern dish, sort of a lamb meatloaf. It is usually served with a mint-flavored yogurt sauce, but is delicious even without it. Coconut yogurt is now available at many health food stores, and would work well with kibbe. Many restaurants make kibbe into small loaves, which are floated in sauce. However, you can use a regular loaf pan if you prefer, and slice it like meat loaf.

1 Preheat oven to 375°F.
2 Combine all ingredients (except pine nuts), and shape into 2 small loaves or 1 large loaf.
3 Sprinkle top with pine nuts and gently press them into the meat. Bake in a 9-inch dish for 30 minutes, or until browned.
4 Serve with rice pilaf.

Makes 1 large loaf or 2 small loaves

World's Easiest Shepherd's Pie

Shepherd's pie has always been a family favorite around our house. It is really easy to make if you use frozen vegetables (which are quick and also retain their nutrients). If you are always in a hurry, here is a trick to remember: Browned ground meat freezes very well for later use. Be sure to drain the fat and let it cool completely before bagging and freezing. Then pull out what you need and throw the meat in your pot or casserole. It works perfectly for this recipe, and makes it a quick meal to put together.

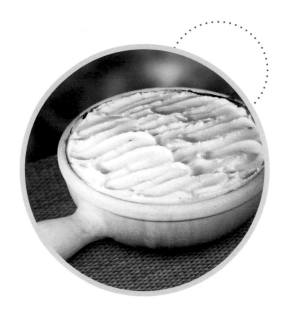

1 Preheat oven to 350°F.

2 Heat oil in a skillet, then cook onion and garlic until soft.

3 Add meat and continue cooking over medium heat, until meat is cooked through.

4 Add vegetables and return the skillet to boiling.

5 Add salsa and cook for an additional 10 minutes.

6 Season with salt and pepper, then pour mixture into a casserole. Top with mashed potatoes.

7 Bake casserole for 35–40 minutes, until top is golden and meat is bubbling.

Makes 4–6 servings

I tablespoon olive oil

I onion, chopped finely

I garlic clove, minced

I pound lean ground meat

I (1-pound) package mixed
   frozen vegetables

I cup GF salsa

4 cups mashed potatoes

Salt and pepper (to taste)

*It is fine to use instant mashed potatoes if you are sure they do not contain additives or preservatives. Barbara's Potatoes are a good choice, and can be made with broth or a dairy substitute of your choice.

Note: If you have non-veggie eaters, put the vegetables in the food processor or blender and puree them before adding to the pot.

Mexican Corn Bread Pizza

1 recipe corn bread
  (see Sweet Corn Bread
  recipe on page 78)
1 pound ground beef
1 onion, chopped
1 teaspoon chili powder
1 teaspoon garlic powder
¼ cup salsa
Salt and pepper (to taste)
1 (8-ounce) package Daiya
  shredded, cheddar-style
  cheese, divided

This is a simple recipe that is easy to throw together. If your child cannot tolerate corn, you can substitute Cream of Rice cereal for cornmeal in this recipe.

1 Preheat oven to 400°F.

2 Prepare corn bread and spread batter in a greased 12-inch pizza pan.

3 Bake cornbread for 8–10 minutes, or until lightly brown.

4 Brown meat and onion in a pan, and then drain. Set aside.

5 Add seasoning to salsa and spoon over cornbread crust.

6 Sprinkle 1 cup "cheese" over baked crust.

7 Top with meat mixture and remaining cheese.

8 Bake cornbread pizza for 4–5 minutes, or until cheese is melted.

Makes 4–6 servings

Veggie Burgers

Rebecca Sullivan is a mom who wrote to me looking for a homemade clay recipe a few years ago. When I sent her the recipe that had appeared in *The ANDI News*, she was so thrilled that she immediately sent me her own recipe for veggie burgers. It has been a big hit with her family, and is a great way to sneak in some lima beans if you are so inclined. Other beans could be substituted. The addition of apple is ingenious, but could be omitted if you are limiting fruits.

1 carrot
1 onion
1 apple, cored, peeled, and sliced (or pear)
2 eggs (or egg replacer and amount liquid suggested)
¼ cup tapioca flour
2 tablespoons potato starch
¼–½ cup water
1 teaspoon parsley
1 teaspoon xanthan gum
½ teaspoon salt
½ pound lima beans, cooked
Oil

1 Place vegetables and fruit in a food processor or blender and process.

2 Add eggs and continue to process until smooth.

3 Add flour, starch, and remaining ingredients (except lima beans) and process to incorporate.

4 Add lima beans to blender and process for 2 minutes or until completely mixed. Add water as needed to form a thick batter.

5 Heat oil in a frying pan, then spoon in batter, forming burger-sized patties.

6 Fry patties until brown on one side, turn and flatten if necessary. Fry until the second side is golden too.

7 Serve with applesauce or fruit relish.

Makes 4–6 servings

Note: If patties appear to flake or crumble while frying, they are too wet. Add more flour.

✴ Bean Burgers

1 cup black beans
   (or kidney beans)
Water
Pinch GF baking soda
1 cup sunflower seeds
4 eggs
½ cup carrots, peeled
   and grated
½ cup kale, finely chopped
½ cup onion, finely chopped
1 tablespoon fresh parsley,
   finely chopped
1 tablespoon rosemary
1 tablespoon basil
1¼ teaspoons salt
Pepper (optional)

This recipe comes from Julie Matthews' excellent book, *Cooking to Heal*. Julie is extremely knowledgeable about dietary interventions of all types, and is an inventive cook. Visit her website at www.nourishinghope.com for more information or to order her book. Like all her recipes, Julie's bean burgers are nutrient-dense and yummy!

1 Expeller-pressed coconut oil, ghee, or other oil

2 Soak beans overnight in water with baking soda.

3 Drain and rinse beans with water.

4 Place beans in a pot and cover with fresh water.

5 Cook beans on low to medium heat for 20–25 minutes until soft, but not mushy. Do not add salt to the beans while they cook — it will make them tough.

6 Grind sunflower seeds in a blender or food processor until the consistency of nut flour.

7 Remove seeds, then place beans in food processor and process until coarsely chopped.

8 In a bowl, combine beans with the sunflower seed meal, eggs, carrots, kale, onion, herbs, and seasonings.

9 Knead mixture with your hands until mixed thoroughly.

10 Form mixture into patties and fry in a skillet with oil. Cook on medium for at least 10 minutes on each side.

11 These burgers can be kept refrigerated for up to 3 days. They can be eaten room temperature or reheated in the oven or on the stove. Cooked patties freeze well.

Makes 4–6 servings

✺ Buckwheat Burgers

Anyone who knows me knows that I love, love, love kasha. I grew up on the stuff, and I could eat it every day. For some, it seems to be an acquired taste, but if your family does not typically eat buckwheat groats, try them. They have fiber and B vitamins, and make a great substitute for other grains. **Note**: When making kasha for a pilaf, you should coat in egg and cook them in a dry pan before adding liquid. This keeps the grains individual and gives them a wonderful nutty flavor. For this recipe, however, you want to forgo that step so that the "burger" will hold together nicely.

⅔ cup water (or broth)

Salt

⅓ cup coarse kasha (whole grains or coarse granulation)

5–6 large portobello mushrooms (if tolerated)

1 cup onion

1 cup bell pepper, seeded

¼ cup olive oil, divided

2 garlic cloves, finely chopped

½ teaspoon pepper

3 tablespoons fresh parsley

1 egg, beaten

1 teaspoon GF Worcestershire sauce

1½ cups GF bread crumbs, divided

1 Bring salted water to a boil in a heavy saucepan, then stir in kasha.

2 Return to a boil, and then lower heat to a simmer.

3 Cover and cook kasha until water is absorbed, about 10 minutes.

4 Transfer kasha to a bowl, and allow to cool.

5 Put mushrooms in a food processor or blender and blitz until finely chopped.

6 Sauté onions and peppers in 1 tablespoon oil until soft. Add chopped mushrooms, garlic, 1 teaspoon salt, and pepper. Cook until all mushroom liquid cooks off, about 10 minutes. (If your children think they hate vegetables, put the mixture back into the blender or food processor and blend until it is very fine.)

7 Transfer this mixture to the bowl of kasha and mix in parsley, egg, and Worcestershire. Add bread crumbs and mix well.

8 Form mixture into patties, cover with plastic wrap, and chill for at least 1 hour.

9 Heat oil in a heavy 12" pan. Fry patties, turning only once, until golden on each side (about 5 minutes total).

Makes 4–6 servings

Nadine's Outrageous Tuna (Or Chicken) Casserole

Pasta

1 (12 ounce or 16-ounce) package GFCF pasta

Cold water

2 (5-ounce) cans CF chunk light tuna in water, drained (or chicken)

1 (16-ounce) package Imagine Portobello Mushroom Soup

1½ cups frozen mixed vegetables

Sauce

4 tablespoons GFCF margarine

4 tablespoons sweet rice flour

2 cups milk substitute (preferably almond or DariFree™)

If you have been to an Autism Research Institute conference, you have probably met Nadine Gilder. In addition to being a certified nutrition counselor, Nadine is a great cook! Since her 20-year-old son is on a GFCF and soy-free diet, she has had a lot of practice. The Gilders love tuna casserole, so Nadine came up with a good duplicate that uses no gluten or casein. Since many autism specialists are now suggesting our children eat **no fish** due to the very high levels of mercury, feel free to substitute chicken. If you need help for your child or taking care of yourself, Nadine can be reached through her website, www.EvolutionLifestyleandNutrition.com). The Gilders think that the recipe is outrageously good, hence its name.

For the Pasta:

1 Cook pasta until it is al dente, then drain and rinse with water.

2 In a separate bowl, mix together tuna, soup, and vegetables.

For the Sauce:

1 Preheat oven to 350°F.

2 Melt margarine in a small saucepan over low to medium heat. Add flour and blend (with a fork or spoon) into a paste. Add milk substitute gradually while stirring.

3 Stir sauce and cook over medium heat until smooth and thick.

4 Pour white sauce gently over pasta mixture to distribute evenly over the pasta.

5 Transfer mixture to a 9"x 13" pan, taking care not to mash the pasta.

6 Bake for 45–60 minutes, until the mixture is thoroughly warmed and bubbling on top.

Makes 4–6 servings

Optional: You can add GFCF bread crumbs or cornflakes on top for a crispy topping.

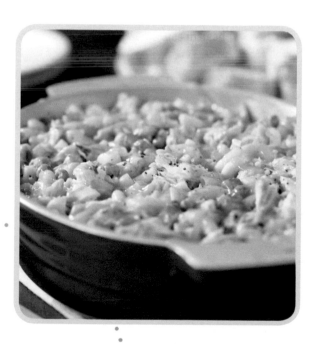

Grilled Pork Tenderloin

2 (1-pound) pork tenderloins
(they usually come two to
a package)
¼ cup oil
¼ cup rice wine vinegar
½ cup GF tamari sauce
½ cup cooking sherry
1 tablespoon lemon juice
1 teaspoon grated ginger
1 teaspoon sesame oil

 If you like, you can bring marinade to a boil and then gently boil for at least 10 minutes until you have a thick sauce to serve with meat. (Do not use marinade unless it has been cooked for at least 10 minutes.)

Pork tenderloin is a versatile cut of meat. It is easy to prepare, and adapts to many recipes. It can be expensive; watch for specials and buy several when they are on sale. They freeze well if properly wrapped, and defrost overnight in the fridge. When you cook them outside, you avoid heating up your kitchen, and the smokiness of the barbecue adds a lot of flavor. While you can rub with olive oil and spices and toss it on the grill, I like to marinate tenderloin for a few hours (or overnight), and then cook it. You can marinate in a large zippered plastic bag, and every time you go into the refrigerator, give it a turn! Any marinade will work (remember, I said it is versatile), but here is one with an Asian touch to get you started. The same marinade and technique works well for a boneless pork roast, but it will take longer to cook as it is thicker.

1 Combine all ingredients in a large bag.
2 Marinate pork for 4 hours or overnight.
3 Heat grill and remove pork from marinade.
4 Cook for 18–20 minutes, turning every 5 minutes. The internal temperature should reach 155°F.
5 Cover meat with foil, and let rest for 10 minutes.

Makes 4–6 servings

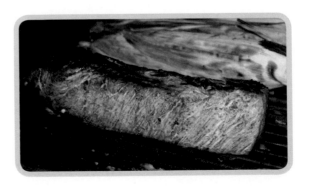

Basic Pork Tenderloin

Pork tenderloin can be grilled, stuffed, or just roasted in the oven. I like to buy these when they are on special and put them in the freezer. I also buy turkey "tenderloins," which can be prepared in the same manner as their porcine counterparts.

1 Preheat oven to 425°F.

2 Brown pork in a large pan and remove to a platter.

3 In same pan, sauté onions and garlic in oil for 5 minutes. Add pears and cook for 2 minutes more.

4 Add broth, vinegar, and mustard, and stir well. Add salt and pepper.

5 Place pork in a baking pan and cover with cooked mixture.

6 Cover with foil and bake for 30–60 minutes — meat thermometer should read 170°F for fully cooked pork.

7 Let rest for 10 minutes before slicing.

8 Serve with gravy and potatoes or rice.

Makes 4–6 servings

1 (3-pound) pork tenderloin

2 cups onion, chopped

3 garlic cloves, peeled and chopped

3 tablespoons olive oil

2 tart, firm-fleshed pears

¾ cup chicken broth

2 tablespoons apple cider vinegar

1 teaspoon prepared mustard

Salt and pepper (to taste)

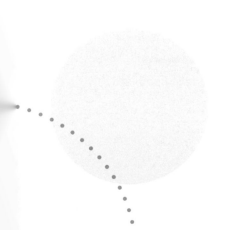

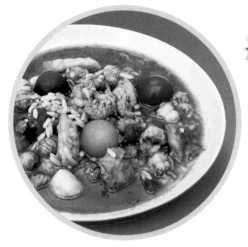

Cioppino

Trader Joe's makes a wonderful fish stew, available in their freezer section. I always doctor it with a little red wine and fresh garlic, and then add some extra shrimp to stretch it. I serve it in bowls over rice or noodles. If you are not lucky enough to have a TJ's in your neighborhood, it is not hard to make. It is a forgiving recipe...tinker at will! The alcohol will give a lovely flavor but will "cook out," so it is fine for the whole family. Traditionally this is made with fresh clams and mussels, but I always buy frozen. If you are up for it, scrub and cook your own shellfish.

3 tablespoons olive oil

1 medium onion, chopped

2 garlic cloves, minced

3 tablespoons fresh parsley
    leaves, minced

1 (26-ounce) container Pomi
    chopped tomatoes, with juice

1 (6.5-ounce) can minced
    clams, in juice

1 bay leaf

1 tablespoon dried basil

½ teaspoon dried thyme

½ teaspoon dried oregano

1½ cups dry red wine

½ pound frozen mussels

½ pound frozen clams

1–2 dozen shrimp, cleaned
    and deveined

½ pound scallops

1 pound fish fillets
    (halibut, cod, or scrod),
    cut into bite-sized chunks

Salt and freshly ground pepper
    (to taste)

1 Heat olive oil, then add onion, garlic, and parsley to a large soup pot or cast-iron Dutch oven over medium-low heat.

2 Cook slowly, stirring occasionally, until onions are soft and translucent.

3 Add tomatoes with juice, minced clams, herbs, and wine; bring just to a boil, then reduce heat to low, cover, and simmer 45–60 minutes. The sauce should be soupy; if it gets too thick, add a little wine or water.

4 Stir in frozen clams, mussels, shrimp, scallops, and fish fillets. Cover and simmer 5–7 minutes until shrimp and whitefish are opaque and shellfish is heated through. If you are using fresh shellfish, they should open in 5–7 minutes. Throw away any that do not open.

5 Do not overcook or the fish will get tough. Remove and discard bay leaf; season with salt and pepper.

6 Remove from heat and ladle broth and seafood into large soup bowls.

Makes 8 servings

✳ Almond-Crusted Fish

Ground nuts make a great breading for fish. Nuts give the fish a lovely crunch and add protein and healthy oils. Visit the Monterey Bay Aquarium website at www. montereybayaquarium.org to download their Seafood Watch list; it is a regional guide for good seafood choices. Pick a firm-fleshed fish from the "Best Choice" or "Good Alternative" list; this will differ depending on where you live.

½ cup blanched almonds,
   processed to fine texture
¼ cup GF flour
1 teaspoon salt
½ teaspoon pepper
2 eggs
4 (6-ounce) fish filets
3 tablespoons olive oil

1 Combine almonds, flour, and seasonings in a shallow bowl.

2 Place eggs in a separate bowl and beat.

3 Dredge fish in eggs, then nut/flour mixture.

4 Fry fish in hot oil until golden, about 4 minutes on each side.

5 If desired, fry a handful of slivered almonds in hot oil, and scatter over fish.

Makes 4 servings

Schnitzel

1 (1-pound) pork tenderloin
1 egg
1 cup GFCF bread crumbs
   (I prefer GF panko)
½ teaspoon salt
½ teaspoon pepper
½ teaspoon garlic powder
2 tablespoons oil

Weiner schnitzel is typically made with veal, but pork tenderloin makes an excellent, simple dish. It is easy to prepare, and is versatile. You can use veal if you prefer.

1 Cut pork tenderloin crosswise into approximately 8 slices.

2 Place each slice between 2 sheets of plastic wrap, and gently pound pork with a rolling pin until about ¼" thick.

3 Place egg in a shallow bowl and beat.

4 Place bread crumbs in a pie pan, and season with salt, pepper, and garlic powder.

5 Heat oil in a large skillet over medium-high heat until hot.

6 Dip each pork piece in egg, then dip in crumb mixture to coat.

7 Place coated pork slices into hot oil and cook about 3 minutes on each side, until golden.

Makes 8 servings

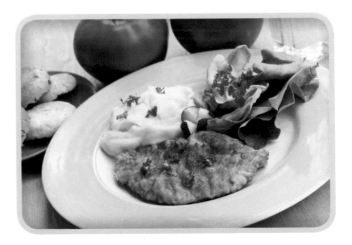

Hungarian Goulash

There is a big difference between imported sweet paprika and the domestic stuff, which really just makes food red. Be sure to buy the real thing when making goulash. This recipe uses beef chuck, but you can upgrade to a nicer cut of beef or veal cubes. This dish is delicious served with noodles and, if soy is tolerated, mock sour cream.

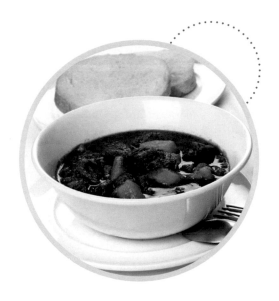

1 Add approximately ½ teaspoon salt to meat. Brown meat in oil, then add onions and paprika.

2 Let meat simmer in its own juice, along with paprika and bay leaf, for about 1 hour on low heat.

3 Add water, potatoes, pepper, and remaining salt.

4 Cover and simmer until potatoes are done and meat is tender.

5 Remove and discard bay leaf, and serve.

Makes 4–6 servings

1 teaspoon salt, divided
2 pounds beef chuck, cut into 1" cubes
2 tablespoons olive oil
2 onions, chopped
2 tablespoons imported sweet paprika
1 bay leaf
4 cups water
4 potatoes, peeled and diced
¼ teaspoon black pepper

Pork Stew

2½ pounds assorted Latin root
    vegetables (e.g., malanga,
    yucca, boniato, true yam)
Water
2 tablespoons safflower oil
1 pound boneless pork loin,
    trimmed of fat and cut into
    ½" cubes
Salt and freshly ground black
    pepper (to taste)
1 onion, diced
2 tablespoons garlic, minced
1 tablespoon imported sweet
    paprika
2 teaspoons ground cumin
1 teaspoon red or green chili,
    minced
2 quarts chicken stock
1 lime, juiced

When I began working at home, I had more time to spend shopping, and often explored new neighborhoods and stores. In one store, I found many exotic root vegetables. After doing a bit of research, I realized that these roots, while exotic to me, are everyday fare in many Latino communities. They are inexpensive, and are a nice change from potatoes. They are also great for people on rotating diets.

1 Peel root vegetables (if using yucca or true yams, take care to peel off bitter under layer).

2 Dice root vegetables and set aside in a large bowl. Fill with water to cover.

3 Heat oil over medium-high heat in a large pan.

4 Sprinkle pork with salt and pepper; add to pan and brown on all sides, 5–7 minutes. Remove pork and set aside.

5 Drain all but 1 tablespoon fat from pan, add onion, and sauté over medium heat, stirring occasionally. Cook until translucent, about 5–7 minutes.

6 Add garlic, spices, and chilies, and sauté 1 minute more.

7 Add stock and root vegetables, and bring just to a boil.

8 Reduce heat to very low, and simmer, stirring occasionally, for about 30 minutes or until pork is tender and vegetables are easily pierced with a fork.

9 Stir in lime juice and serve.

Makes 4–6 servings

Veal Stew

My friend Annie gave me this recipe years ago. It came from her mother, Judith Williams, and it is delicious. If soy is not tolerated, you can omit the mock sour cream. Though it will be a much different dish, it will still be good. You could also use a non-dairy yogurt such as coconut.

1 Sauté onions in oil. Stir in veal, and brown on all sides.

2 Add remaining ingredients (except Sour Supreme).

3 Cover and cook over low heat until meat is tender.

4 Add Sour Supreme when meat is fully cooked, and cook gently until heated through.

5 Serve with GF noodles.

Makes 4–6 servings

1 large onion, chopped

Oil

3 pounds veal

1½ cups Tofutti Sour Supreme*(or non-dairy yogurt)

¼–½ cup white wine

½ cup mushrooms, chopped

3 tablespoons imported sweet paprika

Sour Supreme now comes in a non-hydrogenated version. If you use soy products, you should try to find this version.

Beef Stew

⅓ cup GF flour blend
   (or sweet rice flour)
1 teaspoon salt
1 teaspoon imported sweet
   paprika
¼ teaspoon black pepper
2 pounds top round beef,
   cubed
¼ cup oil (to cut fat, use a
   non-stick pan with oil spray)
2 cups water
1 small onion, peeled and
   chopped
6 very small onions, peeled
   (fresh or frozen pearl onions
   work well)
6 carrots, peeled and cut into
   small chunks
6 medium potatoes, cut into
   chunks
6 fresh beets, peeled and cut
   in half
1 cup fresh green beans,
   snapped and halved

This is my friend Barbara Crooker's recipe. It is very tasty, but of course some children will not touch stew. You may be surprised, however, and it is worth trying. My son loves anything with meat in it, and has even come to eat the vegetables without making a fuss. Add any vegetables you like: try frozen if fresh are not available.

1 Place flour, salt, paprika, and pepper in a bag. Then shake beef cubes in mixture.

2 Heat oil in a Dutch oven, add beef and brown.

3 Pour in water and onions.

4 Bring to a boil then reduce heat and simmer for 2 hours.

5 Add remaining vegetables and cook 40 minutes more. If using frozen vegetables (e.g., peas, corn), add them only for last 5 minutes.

Makes 4–6 servings

Easy Corned Beef and Cabbage

I am hardly Irish, but this is great for St. Patrick's day or any day. If you think your child will not touch vegetables, puree them in the blender first.

1 In a deep sauté pan with lid, heat broth, garlic, caraway seeds, and pepper to boiling.
2 Add cabbage and potatoes, then reduce to a simmer. Cook until potatoes are tender.
3 Remove pan from heat. Add corned beef to the vegetables, and heat through.

Makes 4–6 servings

1 (14-ounce) can GF vegetable or chicken broth
2 garlic cloves, peeled and sliced
½ teaspoon caraway seeds
¼ teaspoon coarsely ground black pepper
1 small cabbage head, cored and chopped
1 pound baby potatoes (peeling is optional)
¾ pound thin-sliced deli corned beef*

Be sure to read label on corned beef; it often contains forbidden ingredients. If possible, buy corned beef and other luncheon meats that are kosher for Passover — they contain no corn and will usually be additive-free.

Stir-Fried Pork

2 tablespoons olive oil

4 cups onion, sliced vertically

1 cup broccoli florets, chopped
finely

1 pork tenderloin, cut into thin
slices

1 red bell pepper, chopped

½ cup green onions, chopped

1 tablespoon sugar (optional)

1 tablespoon fresh ginger,
peeled and minced

3 garlic cloves, minced

½ cup chicken broth

3 tablespoons GF soy sauce
(or tamari sauce)

½ cup dry-roasted cashews,
chopped (or almonds)

2 teaspoons sesame oil

2 cups hot, cooked
long-grain rice

Here is another way to use pork tenderloin. It is tasty, and you can use it to slip in some veggies. If you are lucky, your children will not even notice. Sliced beef or chicken also make great stir-fry dinners. If you want, you can use frozen veggies.

1 Place a wok or large nonstick skillet on medium-high heat. Add olive oil and onion, and when hot, cook 8 minutes, stirring occasionally.

2 Remove onion from pan and place in a bowl.

3 Add broccoli to pan; stir-fry 3 minutes. Remove broccoli and add it to onions.

4 Cook pork and pepper, stirring for 5 minutes, or until meat loses its pink color.

5 Reduce heat. Stir in green onions, sugar, ginger, and garlic, and cook 30 seconds, stirring constantly.

6 Stir in onion mixture, chicken broth, soy sauce, and cashews; cook 1 minute.

7 Drizzle with sesame oil and serve with rice.

Makes 4–6 servings

Salmon Burgers

When I was a child, my mother made these and called them salmon patties. We used to groan when she made them — it was never a favorite. But one night, when I was desperate for something to cook, I found a can of salmon in my pantry and thought, "Why not?" To my surprise, my children and my husband loved them. I have to admit that they tasted a lot better than I remembered. Although children do not usually love fish, this may be an exception, and salmon adds calcium and essential fatty acids to the diet.

1 Use a fork to break up salmon as much as possible. Either remove little bones or crush with your fingers — they are soft and edible, and add calcium.
2 Add egg and seasonings, and mix well. Add just enough breading mix to keep the mixture together, and form as you would for burgers.
3 Heat about ¼" oil in a 10" frying pan; you do not need a lot of oil. When oil is quite hot, place burgers in pan, leaving enough space between them to turn easily.
4 Fry burgers on each side until well browned and forming a crispy outer surface.
5 Place burgers on a paper towe-lined plate and blot off excess oil.
6 Keep warm and serve like burgers.

Makes 4–6 servings

1 (14-ounce) can salmon, drained
1 egg, lightly beaten (you may omit if egg is not tolerated)
Salt, pepper, and seasonings of your choice (to taste)
½ cup GF breading mix or ground GF crackers*
Oil

*If avoiding grains or starches, you can use ground nut meal. A simple filler can be made by whirring GF crackers in a food processor or blender. I especially like Blue Diamond nut crackers, which come in several varieties. (Read the ingredients carefully as some varieties contain milk.)

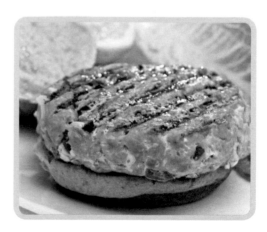

Salmon Puffs

1 (14-ounce) can salmon,
   drained
½ cup GF breading mix
   (more if fish is pureed)
2 tablespoons onion, grated
1 tablespoon lemon juice
Pepper (to taste)
1 egg
½ cup milk substitute
1½ teaspoons GF baking
   powder
Salt (to taste)*

 Because salmon tends to be salty, I never add salt to this recipe. If you want, add ½–1 teaspoon salt.

These are a light, tasty way to get some protein and calcium into your child. This dish is so much like the previous recipe that I almost left it out. I decided to include both recipes because some children may go for the fattier version and reject this recipe, which is baked. There is no reason you could not substitute crab or tuna for the salmon, and any of them would make a nice lunch or a light dinner. For a really smooth puff, put the mixture in a food processor or blender until smooth, and then proceed.

1 Preheat oven to 350°F.
2 Remove visible bones and skin from salmon (optional).
3 Add remaining ingredients in a bowl, and mix by hand or process until smooth.
4 Form into small round balls, and place on a cookie sheet sprayed with cooking spray.
5 Bake puffs for 25–30 minutes, or until brown. These puffs get very crispy on the outside, but remain soft inside.

Makes 4–6 servings

Mom's Cassoulet

Ok, so Mom is not really French, and this is not a truly authentic cassoulet. The real thing calls for all kinds of fancy (and expensive) ingredients, and takes days to cook. But this recipe is delicious, fairly easy, and makes a wonderful meal on a cold winter day. It has so many different things in it that everyone will find something they like, even if it means picking a little. Mom says, "Try it, it is worth the trouble." If you prefer, cook the beans the day before, and refrigerate them until you are ready to prepare the dish.

1 Preheat oven to 250°F.

2 Brown lamb in a little oil.

3 Remove lamb and brown chicken, then remove chicken and brown sausage.

4 Brown onions and garlic in same pan over low heat. Cook until very dark and set aside.

5 Cook beans according to package directions, but cook them until they are almost, but not completely, done.

6 In a large casserole or Dutch oven, layer lamb, sausage, chicken, onions, and beans.

7 Pour wine over mixture. Sprinkle top with parsley and toss in bay leaf.

8 Cover tightly and bake for about 4 hours. Most of liquid should be gone, and meat and beans will be soft.

9 Remove and discard bay leaf, add salt and pepper, and serve.

Makes 4–6 servings

1 pound lean lamb, cut into chunks

Olive oil (or safflower oil)

1 pound chicken, boned, skinned, and cut into chunks

½ pound GF sausage, cut into chunks (with no preservatives)

2 onions, sliced

2 garlic cloves

½ pound white beans

2 cups red wine

1–3 parsley sprigs, chopped

1 bay leaf

Salt and pepper (to taste)

"Mexican" Casserole

1 pound ground beef

1 onion, chopped

1 (6-ounce) can black olives, sliced

1 (15-ounce) can GF refried beans* (dehydrated refried beans are excellent)

1 (10-ounce) jar GF salsa, divided

1 (3-ounce) can mild green chilies, chopped

1 (8-ounce) package cheddar-style Daiya, divided

CF sour cream substitute (if soy is tolerated)

GF tortilla chips (if corn is tolerated)

 *Canned refried beans are widely available and come in non-fat versions (many brands have lard in them — besides being high in saturated fat, lard generally has a good amount of artificial preservatives). Check your health food store for dehydrated beans. They reconstitute with boiling water and taste very good. They also come in a black bean variety, and these make an excellent casserole too.

I am sure this recipe did not originate south of the border, but it is very good and a real winter favorite at our house. My mother uses it as an appetizer with chips, but I have always served it as a main course, with a salad and tortilla chips. It is one of my son's favorite dishes.

1 Preheat oven to 350°F.

2 Brown beef and onion, and drain well. Stir in olives.

3 In a 2-quart casserole, spread refried beans to cover bottom.

4 Over beans, spoon half the beef mixture. Add half the salsa. Sprinkle half the Daiya cheese on top of casserole.

5 Place chilies over the cheese, and then cover with other half of meat. Cover meat with remaining salsa.

6 Top with remaining Daiya cheese, then top with 4–5 tablespoons CF sour cream substitute.

7 Bake casserole for 25-30 minutes, until whole casserole is bubbling.

8 Serve with tortilla chips.

Makes 4–6 servings

Mexican Casserole with Chicken Variation:
An excellent variation of this recipe uses chopped, cooked chicken breast in place of ground beef. I use green salsa, which can generally be found at the grocery store (look in the Mexican food section). If you cannot find green salsa, red is also acceptable.

Sloppy Joes

Most children like sloppy joes. This is a dish I had completely forgotten about until my husband revived it one night when he took charge of dinner. My children usually eat it with a spoon, rather than as a sandwich, because they think it is too messy. You can certainly try it over an appropriate bread or bun if you prefer. This just barely qualifies as a recipe, but Serge swears this is the best way to make it. I use Heinz organic ketchup, which has very few ingredients.

1 Brown beef, garlic, and onion, and drain off fat.
2 To meat mixture, add ketchup, Worcestershire sauce, and brown sugar. Cook on low heat until mixture is the right consistency, some sauce but not too wet, according to your preferences.
3 Keep adding ketchup and Worcestershire sauce to taste. Season with salt and pepper.
4 Serve over GF bread or buns if desired.

Makes 4–6 servings

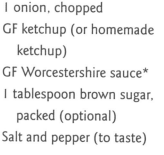

1 pound lean ground beef
1 garlic clove, minced
1 onion, chopped
GF ketchup (or homemade ketchup)
GF Worcestershire sauce*
1 tablespoon brown sugar, packed (optional)
Salt and pepper (to taste)

 *Worcestershire sauce usually contains soy and/or corn products. "Natural flavorings" may or may not be GF. Check with the company, and if a GF form cannot be found, you can substitute another flavorful sauce. Most sauces do contain some soy or corn however, such as wheat-free Tamari or Soy Sauce. Check with the various mail order companies to find a good GF substitute.

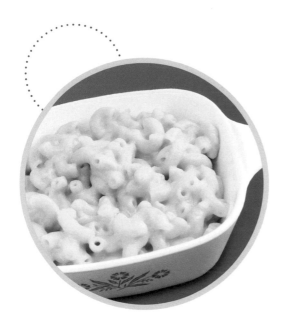

Mock Mac and Cheese

I have never met a child who does not like macaroni and cheese. Unfortunately, both the wheat macaroni and the cheese sauce are forbidden for our kids. Daiya now makes a great cheese substitute, and there are several excellent GF pastas available (e.g., Tinkayada brand). The white sauce (béchamel) used in this recipe can also serve as the base for any creamed casserole or soup.

2 tablespoons CF margarine
2 tablespoons sweet rice flour
1 cup milk substitute
    (soy or potato is preferable)
Salt and pepper (to taste)
½ pound GF macaroni
Water
1 onion, diced
½ (8-ounce) package Daiya
    cheddar-style cheese
2–3 dashes GF Worcestershire
    sauce (optional)
1 tablespoon CF margarine
    (optional)

1 Preheat oven to 350°F.
2 To make a white sauce, melt margarine in a small saucepan.
3 Add flour and blend into a paste. Add milk substitute very gradually, stirring constantly.
4 Continue stirring, add salt, and cook over medium heat until the sauce is smooth and thickened. Set aside.
5 Cook macaroni al dente in a pot with water according to package directions. Drain, rinse, and drain again.
6 Place cooked noodles in a small, ovenproof casserole.
7 Stir in onion, Worcestershire sauce, white sauce, salt, and pepper into noodles. Mix well and dot with CF margarine.
8 Bake for 20–30 minutes.
9 If desired, top with crumbled potato chips, extra grated Daiya, or GF breading mix (into which a little melted CF margarine has been added).

Makes 4–6 servings

Sides

Just about every dinner at our house includes a salad and at least one side. Sometimes this is a cooked vegetable, and sometimes it is a grain or other starch. Many people find it is harder to come up with an inventive, nutritious side than a main course. Hopefully some of these recipes will tempt your family. They include some of my family's favorites.

Some of these "sides" make a good lunch, or an entrée for a light dinner. For dinner, you may want to add a protein source, such as adding leftover meat to a kasha pilaf, or beans to a rice dish. In addition to being a quick-and-easy dinner, using leftovers to accent grains is both nutritious and economical. ★

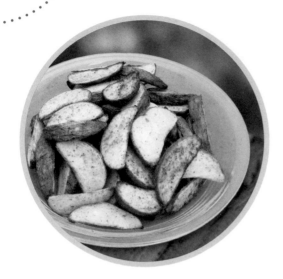

French Fries

There are GF frozen French fries available, though you do have to read the ingredients carefully to make sure they have no wheat. Homemade fries are so special, though, they deserve to be made once in a while. I almost always make frozen fries, but in the summer when we have freshly dug potatoes from our garden, I like to make them from scratch. I slice the potatoes into the shape of chips (i.e., following the shape of the potato) and that is fine with my kids. But if your child will not eat them unless they look right, you might want to invest in one of those gadgets that cuts perfectly shaped fries. Most kitchenware stores carry them, and they are inexpensive. If desired, slice the potatoes as thinly as possible using a mandolin. The result will be the best potato chips you have ever eaten!

Potatoes, peeled and sliced
Oil
Coarse salt (kosher or sea salt)

 Note: *Children need some fat in their diet, but if your child eats predominantly fatty foods, or if the whole family is to eat them, try baking the fries. Spray them with an oil spray, and salt them before they go into a hot (400ºF) oven. Bake until brown. (Timing will depend on the thickness of the fries, so watch carefully.) They are not as delicious or as crispy, but they are very good.*

1 Slice potatoes into shape and thickness desired.
2 Heat about 1½" oil in a deep frying pan. I prefer coconut oil—use whatever is best tolerated by your child.
3 Fry potatoes, flipping as they brown on one side, until brown and crispy on all sides.
4 Place fries on a paper towel–lined plate, draining oil as much as possible.
5 Salt and serve while hot.

Servings will vary.

Caution: Do not stand too close to pan, and be sure little ones are not in the area—the moisture in potatoes really makes oil spatter.

Kasha Pilaf

Kasha is made from buckwheat groats, and is available in the kosher section of most supermarkets. Although the name sounds as if it should have gluten, buckwheat is more closely related to rhubarb than to wheat! Buckwheat flour is sometimes produced in factories that also package wheat flours, and contamination has probably led to the idea that buckwheat products are not safe. However, most companies that make kasha make little else and contamination is not a problem. Call the company if you are unsure. Kasha has a nutty flavor, and makes a wonderful grain to serve alone, or as an ingredient in other recipes.

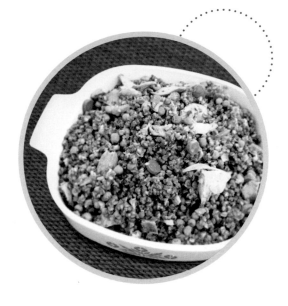

1 Heat oil and cook onion until wilted and soft; add garlic and cook for 2 more minutes.

2 Add kasha, herbs, and seasonings, and stir to coat all grains.

3 Add broth and bring to a boil.

4 Lower heat and cover, simmering 10 minutes or until broth is absorbed and grains are plump.

5 Remove and discard parsley and bay leaf before serving.

Makes 4–6 servings

2 tablespoons olive oil
½ cup onion, chopped
½ teaspoon minced garlic
1 cup kasha
½ teaspoon thyme
2 fresh parsley sprigs
1 bay leaf
Salt and pepper (to taste)
1¾ cups chicken broth
   (or vegetable broth)

Note: Making plain kasha follows the same procedure with two important differences. First, prior to frying the raw grain, a beaten egg is stirred into it. The egg-coated grain is then heated until each grain is separate. At that point, add boiling broth (2 cups water for 1 cup kasha) and stand back, it will spatter! Cover and simmer as above.

The other difference is that onions are the only vegetable added, and salt the only seasoning. Kasha can be used in most recipes that call for cooked rice. Add some small cooked noodles, and you have Kasha Vamishkes. It is an excellent complement to roast beef—my favorite way to serve it is to cut the meat into bite-sized chunks and mix it with cooked Kasha and gravy made from the juice of the roast (use sweet rice flour instead of wheat flour for gravy). Mix in any vegetables you cooked with the beef.

✸new Butternut Squash "Fries"

1 butternut squash
Olive oil
Coarse salt

OK, these are not really fries because they are made in the oven. They are delicious though, and a good source of lots of healthy vitamins. They are so easy to make that there is no excuse not to try them. In fact, the only hard part about this recipe is peeling the squash!

1 Preheat oven to 425°F.
2 With a good vegetable peeler or a very sharp knife, peel squash.
3 Cut squash in half and scoop out seeds and any stringy bits. Cut squash into "fry" shapes, either strips or chips.
4 Place fries on a baking sheet. Brush with oil, or spray with non-stick olive oil spray, and salt generously.
5 Bake for 40 minutes, turning fries after 20 minutes. When fries crisp up and start to brown, they are done.

Makes 4–6 servings

Baked Onion Rings

Onion rings lack the universal appeal of fries, but many children will adore these. I am not sure my son, Sam, really knows what they are, but they are crispy and he thinks they are great. The adults at your table will think these onions are pretty great, too. Since they are baked, they are not too fatty or heavy. Use sweet onions, such as Vidalias, when possible. Purple onions also work well.

1–3 sweet onions
1–2 egg whites (or egg substitute and suggested amount liquid)
2 cups GF breading mix
Salt and pepper (to taste)

1 Preheat oven to 375°F.
2 Slice onions into ¼" rings.
3 Place egg whites in a shallow pan; place breading mix in another shallow pan.
4 Dip each ring in egg white, and then dredge in the breading mixture.
5 Place rings on a baking sheet sprayed with cooking spray. Spray the breaded onions, too.
6 Bake for 12–15 minutes or until crispy and golden brown.

Servings will vary.

 For this recipe, add some crushed GF cornflakes to the breading if tolerated.

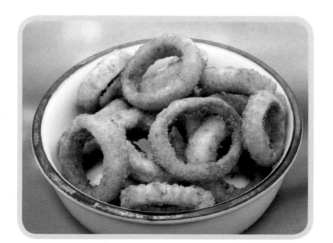

Risotto

4¾ cups GF vegetable or
   chicken stock
½ cup Japanese rice wine
   (alcohol cooks out)
1½ tablespoons olive oil
½ pound Arborio rice
1 onion, chopped
1 garlic clove, minced
1 tablespoon fresh basil,
   chopped (or ½ tablespoon
   dried basil)
1 teaspoon salt
½ teaspoon pepper

Optional Ingredients
Sliced mushrooms (not for
   yeast-free diet)
Peppers, finely chopped
Pitted, sliced black olives
1¾ cups corn kernels, thawed
   or freshly cut from cob

Long a favorite in Italian homes, risotto is finding a spot in American kitchens at last. A delicious, creamy form of white rice, risotto can be made with almost any ingredient added. There are even entire cookbooks devoted to variations of this basic dish. It is a little labor intensive since it requires constant attention while it cooks. I think you will find it well worth the effort. Make the rice after the table is set and all other food is ready to serve, so it can be put on the table as soon as it is finished. If it sits, risotto will get sticky.

1 Combine stock and wine in a saucepan, heat to simmer. Set aside.
2 Sauté oil, rice, onion, and garlic in another pan until rice just starts to brown and onion is soft.
3 Begin adding stock, ½ cup at a time. With each addition of liquid, cook while stirring, until the liquid is absorbed. Then add another ½ cup of liquid and continue this process until you have used most of the liquid, and the rice is creamy and soft.
4 Add basil, seasonings, and any optional ingredients. Continue to stir until whole dish is heated through.
5 Adjust seasonings and serve.

Makes 4–6 servings

Indian Rice

I took an Indian cooking class with a few friends last year, and learned how to make several good dishes. The simplest, however, was rice. My family just loves it when I make the rice this way. Be sure to buy a good, Indian long-grain rice. We like it so much that I always make a large recipe and serve it at more than one dinner. Because of the spices, leftovers also make fantastic rice pudding with almond or coconut milk.

1 Heat oil in a pot over high heat. Add cumin seeds to the hot oil—if the oil is hot enough, seeds will pop a little.

2 After 1 minute, add rice and stir until well coated. Add cinnamon, cardamom, and cloves, and then add water.

3 Bring to a boil, lower heat, and cover. Simmer for about 20 minutes, or until all water is absorbed.

4 Remove cinnamon, cardamom, and cloves. Stir in garam masala and salt.

Makes 4–6 servings

1 tablespoon olive oil
1 teaspoon cumin seeds
2 cups long-grain rice, rinsed
1 cinnamon stick
2–3 green cardamom pods
2–3 whole cloves
4 cups water
1 teaspoon garam masala*
salt (to taste)

Garam masala is an Indian spice blend that can be found in Indian markets and the ethnic food section of some grocery stores.

✹ Bombay Rice

1½ cups water
½ cup orange juice
1 cup rice
⅓ cup raisins
⅓ cup unsweetened, shredded
   coconut
⅓ cup nuts, chopped
   (optional)

This is a slightly sweet side that children (and adults)
will love.

1 Bring water and juice to a boil, then add rice
and raisins.
2 Lower heat, cover, and simmer until liquid is
absorbed, about 20 minutes.
3 Stir in coconut and nuts just before serving.

Makes 4–6 servings

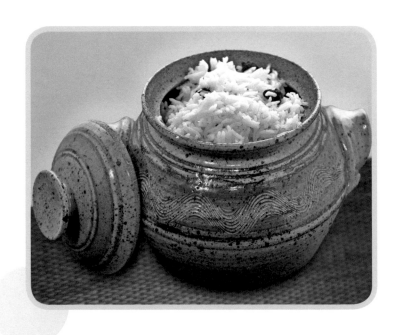

✳ Easiest Rice

Sometimes you just need a dish to be quick!

1 Place all ingredients in a microwave-safe casserole.
2 Cover and microwave on high for 12 minutes.
3 Leave covered for 20–30 minutes. The residual steam will continue cooking, so do not uncover too soon.

Makes 4–6 servings

3½ cups water
2 cups rice
1 tablespoon olive oil
Salt (to taste)

Riz Cous

When we still ate wheat, couscous was one of my son's very favorite foods. I would add some cubed cooked chicken and a few vegetables, and it was a meal he loved. It cooks quickly and is very tasty, and we ate it far more often than rice. I was thrilled when Lundberg Family Farms began selling Riz Cous, a rice-based version, and devastated when it disappeared from my grocery shelves. An e-mail to the company revealed that the product had been discontinued! All was not lost though, since Ms. Karen Skupowski, a Lundberg employee, told me how to make Riz Cous for myself. It is fairly easy to do, and worth a little trouble. You can make a lot of the dry Riz Cous, storing it in an airtight container, to be cooked and used as needed.

I published this recipe in 1998, and was surprised to see it being published in a magazine last year under the name of another (well-known) author. Maybe she called Lundberg, too! In any event, it is a very convenient thing to have in your pantry.

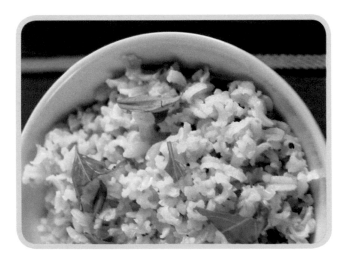

Roasted Rice

1 Preheat oven to 350°F.

2 Grind desired amount of rice in a blender or food processor. The resulting rice should look like tiny pebbles — do not reduce to a powder.

3 Place ground rice on a flat baking sheet, and roast for about 30 minutes.

4 You want it to brown but not burnt. You will need to keep a close watch and stir it several times. This process releases the oils in the rice, and is absolutely necessary for making a product similar to couscous.

5 Cool and store roasted rice in an airtight jar or other container. It does not need refrigeration.

Brown rice

Riz Cous

1 Combine all ingredients in a saucepan.

2 Stirring occasionally, bring to a boil and immediately reduce heat to a simmer.

3 Simmer just until liquid is barely absorbed.

4 Reduce heat to low, cover, and cook for 5 minutes.

5 Remove from heat and fluff with a fork. Leave uncovered for 5 minutes.

6 Turn into a serving dish and fluff again before serving.

Makes 4–6 servings

1½ cups water

¾ cup roasted rice
(see Roasted Rice Recipe,
above)

1 tablespoon olive oil

½ teaspoon salt

✹ Smashed Cauliflower

Water
1 medium cauliflower head,
    trimmed and cut into
    individual florets
    (or 1 small package frozen
    cauliflower)
2 tablespoons olive oil
Kosher salt
Ground pepper

This is another recipe that will get some veggies into your family — painlessly. This is a great substitute for mashed potatoes, and is a great addition to a holiday meal where there are often many heavy dishes.

1 Bring a large pot of water to boil and add cauliflower. Cook until tender, about 10 minutes.
2 Reserve ¼ cup water, and drain the rest.
3 Puree cauliflower in a food processor or blender, adding cooking liquid and oil a little at a time, until you get the right consistency.
4 Season with salt and pepper and serve.

Makes 4–6 servings

Charlie's Italian Mashed "Potatoes"

I ate this dish at Charlie Fall's house and had to have the recipe. It is a delicious, nutrient-dense dish that makes a great substitution for potatoes. Often people will know they like it, but not know what it is! If your family thinks they do not like beans...do not tell them what this is!

1 In a deep frying pan or pot, gently heat oil and add onion. Sauté until beginning to caramelize.

2 Add garlic to onion, and cook gently for 1 minute or so. Do not brown, as this can make garlic bitter.

3 Add beans to onions. Add some more oil and a dash of water.

4 Cover and cook gently for 5 minutes or so.

5 Take a hand masher and mash beans in pot. Leave chunky if you want, or mash completely if you prefer.

6 Add more water and/or oil to desired consistency.

7 Cook on low for about 30 minutes. Check, stir, and add liquid from time to time.

8 Season with salt, pepper, and splash or three of tamari. This dish keeps well.

Makes 4–6 servings

Olive oil
1 onion, chopped
2 garlic cloves, minced
2 (15.5-ounce) cans cannellini
    beans, drained and rinsed
Water
Sea salt
Fresh cracked pepper
GF tamari sauce

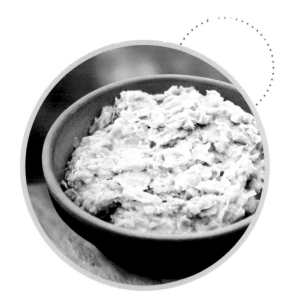

✴ *new* Gingery Carrots

1½ pounds carrots, peeled
  and grated
1 tablespoon cider vinegar
3 tablespoons water
1 teaspoon fresh ginger, grated
1 teaspoon cinnamon
1 tablespoon olive oil
Dash nutmeg (use fresh if
  possible)
Salt and pepper (to taste)

Carrots are so sweet that many children like them (if you can get them to try). This recipe really brings out the natural sweetness of carrots.

1 Preheat oven to 350°F.
2 Place carrots in greased ovenproof casserole.
3 Whisk vinegar, water, ginger, and cinnamon, and stir mixture into carrots.
4 Drizzle with oil, and add salt and pepper.
5 Cover casserole and bake for 40 minutes.

Makes 4–6 servings

✹ Creamy Grits

OK, here is one more "mashed potato switcheroo." This one uses grits, which means those who avoid corn will not be able to enjoy it. If your family can eat corn, however, this is really special and you will love it.

1 Boil water and 2 teaspoons salt in a heavy saucepan and slowly add grits, stirring constantly.

2 Turn heat down to a simmer and cook until grits are thick, about 5 minutes.

3 Stir in coconut milk and oil, and return mixture to a simmer.

4 Cover pan and cook over low heat, stirring occasionally, for 45–50 minutes. The mixture should be very thick and creamy.

5 Remove from heat, and add scallions and Daiya cheese.

6 Add salt and pepper and serve.

Makes 4–6 servings

4 cups water
Salt and pepper (to taste)
1 cup quick-cooking grits
   (not instant)
1 ¼ cups coconut milk
2 tablespoons olive oil
3–4 scallions, chopped
½ cup Daiya or other cheese
   substitute (optional)

Note: This is not a make-ahead recipe, as it will get goopy if it sits too long. Try to finish this off after everything else is ready to go and the table is set.

Rhubarb Applesauce

3 rhubarb stalks
4–5 large organic apples
½ pint organic strawberries
Water
1 teaspoon cinnamon
Sweetener (sugar, stevia,
honey, or lakanto)

Most children love applesauce, and if it is homemade, adults generally like it too. It is often served with latkes for Hanukah, and is always a nice addition to a meal. I have always thought of applesauce as a fall or winter dish, but this version adds some summery fruit. It is different and very good. Use a sweet, rather than a tart, apple variety for this dish.

1 Peel and chop rhubarb. Core, peel, and chop apple. Pick stems off strawberries.
2 Combine all ingredients in a pot, and add water (about ¼ cup) to prevent burning. Once apples begin to cook, they will release more liquid.
3 Cook fruit, covered, over medium heat until boiling, then turn heat down and tilt the cover a little to let steam escape. Stir occasionally.
4 Simmer until most apples have dissolved and mix does not look too watery — around 30 minutes. It is best to turn off the flame while the mix is still a little watery since more water will evaporate while it is cooling down.
5 I prefer the texture when some apple chunks are left in sauce, but you can cook it down or purée in a blender or food processor if you prefer it smooth. If you cannot find rhubarb, try cranberries. You can also use this as a "low-sugar" jam.

Makes 4–6 servings

✳ Pear and Jicama Salad

Jicama (pronounced he-kah-ma) looks like a big brown turnip, but it is actually in the bean family. High in vitamin C and crunch, this "Mexican potato" is often added to salads and vegetable platters. It is great for dipping and stir- fries, and is a great addition to a salad.

1 Combine pears, jicama, and greens in a large serving bowl to make a salad.

2 Blend oil and vinegar in a small bowl, and toss into salad.

3 Add walnuts and seasonings, and serve.

Makes 4–6 servings

3 large firm pears, peeled, cored, and julienned
1 large jicama, peeled and julienned
Salad greens
4 tablespoons walnut oil
2 tablespoons apple cider vinegar
1 cup walnuts, toasted
Salt and pepper (to taste)

Cheap Eats

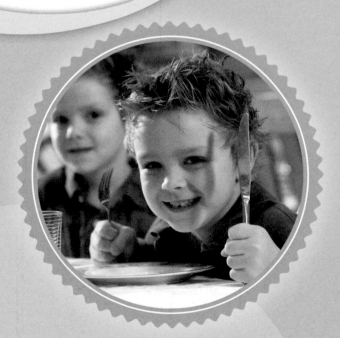

When people meet me or hear me speak, they often come up to tell me why they cannot possibly try dietary intervention for their kids. The reasons are always the same:

"My kid would starve ... he only eats three foods."

"I do not have time to cook" or "I am a terrible cook; I could not possibly do this."

"The rest of my family will not eat these foods, and I do not have time to cook two dinners."

"We are on a limited budget, and we cannot afford a special diet."

Of course, I have answers for all of these excuses, but the last one I take seriously. Many people right now are struggling to put food on the table, and if you add the expense of therapy and special tutors and classes, it is an even bigger challenge.

I do not believe that a special diet necessarily has to be expensive, however. It will get costly if you buy a lot of processed foods to substitute for the foods your children can no longer eat, but most of these are "luxury" items and many are not all that healthy anyway. For example, if cookies are an occasional treat, rather than a daily item, then making some special cookies now and again with a slightly more expensive flour is not really such a big deal.

Here are some of my thoughts on special diets that do not break the bank:

⊙ Make at least one dinner a week a vegetarian meal. You can pack a lot of nutrition into a vegetarian meal while spending less than a dollar per serving.

⊙ Did you know that dried beans cost ⅓ the price of canned beans? There is nothing to cooking your own beans, and if you do a lot at one time, you can freeze them and thaw as you need them.

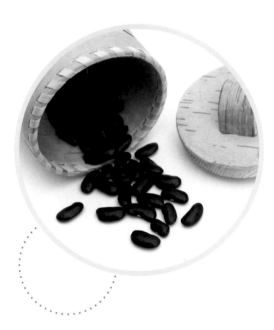

⊙ Soups can be made with all the leftovers you used to throw away. It saves money and can be made into nutritious meals.

⊙ Once or twice a week, use meat as a flavoring element in a dish rather than the main attraction (think Chinese food, which often has a high vegetable-to-meat ratio).

⊙ Make sure that most snacks are one or two ingredients: fruit and CF yogurt, nuts, fresh fruit, vegetable sticks and dip.

⊙ Inexpensive cuts of meat (e.g., skirt steak) are often flavorful, but tough. Marinate overnight and you will greatly tenderize tough cuts and make a great meal for little cash.

⊙ Buy organic for foods that are known to be routinely contaminated; for other produce, buy conventional and use a good vegetable/fruit wash.

This chapter provides a few recipes to get you started on "cheap eats."

Chicken or Fish en Papillote

Cooking in parchment, or *en papillote* as the French say, became all the rage in the 1980s. It is easy to do, allows you to customize each serving, and makes cleanup a breeze. Now I do all my papillote cooking in Reynold's Wrap, which is cheaper and easier to use! It works exactly the same way as parchment, and is a really nice way to make a meal. Because your fish (or chicken) and vegetables are actually steamed, they create a nice little sauce. Be sure to slice all vegetables to about the same thickness so they cook evenly, and open carefully when done cooking!

1 Preheat oven to 450°F.

2 Tear off 1 foil square per meal, approximately 12"x 18".

3 Place each piece of fish in center of a foil square, and brush with oil and juice.

4 Place vegetables on top of fish and season.

5 Fold foil over the food, and seal it up all the way around so that you have an enclosed pouch. Be sure the foil packet is large enough to allow for air to circulate. It will expand as the cooked food gives off steam.

6 If you are using different vegetables, seasonings or condiments, mark each packet with marker, then place them on a baking sheet.

7 Bake for 20–25 minutes (less for fish). When finished, packet will be puffed up quite a bit.

8 Slice packet open carefully, as escaping steam will be very hot.

9 Serve with rice or salad for a quick, nutritious meal.

Makes 1 serving

1 fish filet (or ½ boned, skinned chicken breast)

Onion, thinly sliced

1 potato, thinly sliced (optional)

Assorted vegetables, thinly sliced

1 tablespoon olive oil

1 tablespoon lemon juice (optional, but especially nice with fish)

Condiments of your choice (e.g., salsa, mustard)

Salt, pepper, and any seasoning you like (to taste)

 Note. *You can also cook these on the grill if you prefer.*

Crispy Baked Drumsticks

3 pounds chicken drumsticks
1 teaspoon salt
½ teaspoon paprika
½ cup GF cracker crumbs
1 egg, beaten with 1
    tablespoon water*

 If your child cannot eat eggs, use ¼ cup melted CF margarine to dip chicken in, or use a milk substitute.

Chicken drumsticks are often available in "family packs," and they are always cheap. Most children enjoy picking up drumsticks and like eating with their fingers when Mom gives the OK. This version is low in fat, since it is not fried. If your child is on a SCD or another low-carb diet, use ground nuts for breading.

1 Preheat the oven to 425°F.
2 Remove skin from drumsticks or breast meat.
3 Add spices to crumbs and place in a plate or pie pan. Put egg in a second pie pan.
4 Dip drumsticks first in egg, and then coat thoroughly with breading.
5 Arrange on a foil-lined cookie sheet sprayed with cooking spray.
6 Bake until done, for about 45 minutes.

Makes 4 servings

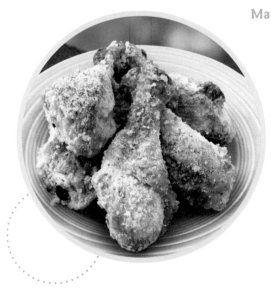

Fried Rice

This recipes works great with leftover chicken, beef, or pork. Note that fresh rice will not absorb the other flavors as well as day-old, but make fresh if you must. Using brown rice will up the nutrition in this dish.

1 In a wok or deep frying pan, bring oil to very high heat.
2 Stir-fry garlic and scallions.
3 Add chicken and then rice, and mix thoroughly.
4 Add tamari and mix well.
5 Sprinkle on sesame oil and serve immediately.

Makes 4 servings

2 tablespoons safflower oil
Fresh vegetables (or package
    frozen mixed vegetables)
2 tablespoons minced garlic
1 teaspoon ginger
1–2 scallions, chopped
2 cups leftover chicken, cubed
4 cups cooked rice
    (day-old is best)
2–4 tablespoons GF
    tamari sauce
2–5 drops sesame oil

✳ Tomato Soup

2 teaspoons olive oil

½ cup onion, chopped

2 garlic cloves, chopped

½ teaspoon salt

Pepper (to taste)

3 cups GF vegetable or chicken broth

1 pound tomatoes, diced

½ teaspoon basil

Many children who wouldn't dream of touching a tomato will happily eat tomato soup. This is one of the great mysteries of life, right up there with why do people who hate peas love pea soup, and people who love carrots hate carrot soup? Imponderable!

1 Heat oil and sauté onion until soft, then add garlic. Cook for 1 minute more.

2 Add remaining ingredients and bring to a boil.

3 Turn down heat to low and simmer soup for 15–20 minutes.

4 Allow to cool and then puree in a food processor or blender.

5 Serve hot or cold.

Makes 4 servings

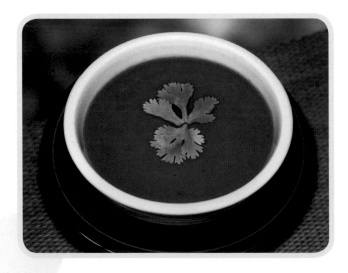

✸ Beans and Rice

Beans and rice is a classic dish. You can vary it in many ways, changing the beans, using brown rice instead of white, using different spices, etc. No matter how you make it, this is a nutritious dish by any standard, and it is inexpensive to make. You can use canned beans, but remember, beans you cook yourself taste great, are low in sodium, and cost *one-fifth* as much!

1 Heat oil in a 2-quart saucepan and sauté onion until soft.

2 Add garlic and cook 1 more minute, then stir in rice.

3 Add broth and bring mixture to a boil.

4 Lower heat and simmer rice for about 20 minutes, covered, until liquid is absorbed.

5 Stir in spices and beans and serve hot.

Makes 4 servings

1 tablespoon olive oil
1 onion, chopped
2 cups water (or broth)
1 cup rice
1 garlic clove , minced
4 cups cooked beans
  (or canned beans)
1 teaspoon cumin
1 tablespoon fresh cilantro,
  chopped (optional)
Salt and pepper (to taste)

Variation: For Caribbean-style rice and beans, add roasted red pepper, 1 teaspoon oregano, 3 drops Tabasco sauce, and 2 tablespoons red wine vinegar. Omit cumin and cilantro.

Holiday Fare

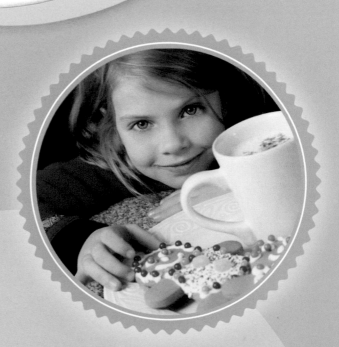

The holiday season—can you remember how exciting it was when you were a child? The season is filled with special events and treats that happen just once a year; most children count the minutes as the holidays draw near.

For families with special needs children, however, the season is very different. All the elements that make the season so exciting for typical children seem to bring out the very worst in children with autism spectrum disorder.

When you rely on predictability to make sense of your world, all the changes in your routine conspire to make this special time of year a disaster. Behaviors you have not seen in months may reappear, and your blood pressure may rise as the temperatures fall. Instead of eager anticipation, you may find yourself filled with dread as the holidays approach.

Even without a special needs child, the holidays can be trying. Anyone who cooks for his or her family knows how stressful holidays can be. Making plans, shopping, and scheduling oven time can cause major headaches. Now add to all this the need to order ahead from specialty food companies and make extra trips to health food stores—is it any wonder that the season seems more trying than joyful?

If ever there is a time when we want to fall back on old eating habits, this is it. Parents may decide to forgo their child's diet because adding special foods to an already full menu is too hard or too expensive. Sometimes parents fear that their child will be missing something wonderful, or perhaps they cannot find good recipes that will make the meal festive.

Tempting as this might be, holidays are definitely not the time to ease up on dietary restrictions. With the stress inherent in the season, why add to it with behavioral regressions made worse by dietary infractions? Instead, plan ahead to maintain the GFCF diet during the holidays, all without sacrificing good food and special treats.

The recipes in this chapter should make it easy to hold your resolve during the holidays. I believe that if you make the GFCF specialties good enough, you can make them instead of your old recipes, rather than adding more to the table.

Most of the recipes that follow were created with Christmas and Thanksgiving in mind, but there are recipes included that would be appropriate for other holidays. Because I was raised in a Jewish home, I have also included several holiday foods modified from recipes I grew up with.

Thanksgiving and Christmas

For many years, we have celebrated Thanksgiving at my sister's apartment in New York. I hate not having Thanksgiving leftovers, however, so I make my own Thanksgiving early in the day. I know, I know... it is a bit much. But we do love Thanksgiving!

You can follow the directions for roasting a big bird in chapter 7, but for holidays, you will also want "the fixings." They are a little tougher to manage, but these are good enough that you should not have to make more than one type of dressing or other side dishes. ★

Twice-Wild Turkey Dressing

½ cup mixed, dried wild
    mushrooms
Water
⅔ cup wild rice
4 teaspoons salt
1 teaspoon CF margarine
2 cups onion, chopped
1 cup celery, finely chopped
¼ cup cooking sherry
Generous pinch of thyme,
    oregano, marjoram, and
    black pepper

Most dressing recipes call for bread: cubed or crumbs.
You can use GF bread for this purpose, but there are
other ways to make dressings that do not require bread
at all.

1 Preheat oven to 350°F.

2 Cover mushrooms with warm water for at least
30 minutes.

3 Remove mushrooms from water, squeeze out as much
excess liquid as possible, and chop well.

4 Rinse rice in cold water.

5 Bring 3 cups water to a boil, then add salt and rice.

6 Return to a boil for 25 minutes, stirring occasionally.
Drain well and set aside.

7 Sauté onion and celery in margarine until slightly
softened.

8 Remove from heat, add remaining ingredients,
and mix well.

9 Bake in a greased casserole for about 1 hour.
(I always make dressing separate from bird as it cooks
more evenly and bird roasts more quickly.)

Makes 4–6 servings

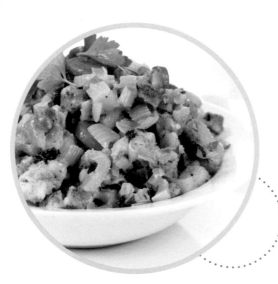

Kasha Dressing

Whenever my birthday falls on a Thursday, it is also Thanksgiving. The first time this happened, I was quite small. Breaking with our usual tradition of Thanksgiving at our house, we instead ate at the home of an aunt and uncle. To this day, I remember that the turkey was stuffed with kasha — my all-time favorite grain, and that my aunt made a cake for me in the shape of a lamb. I have no idea how my aunt made her dressing (or why the cake was made in a lamb mold for that matter!), but this should work if you too love kasha.

4 cups GF chicken or
   vegetable broth
2 eggs, lightly beaten
2 cups kasha, whole or
   coarse grain
2 tablespoons olive oil or
   CF margarine
¼ cup cooking sherry or
   another dry wine
Turkey giblets
2 onions, chopped
1–2 garlic cloves, minced
¼ cup pecans, chopped
   (optional)

1 Preheat oven to 350°F.

2 Bring broth to a boil in a pot, and set aside.

3 Stir eggs into kasha, then cook in a large, deep (greased) frying pan over medium high heat until each grain is separate. Stir carefully to prevent burning and to break apart any clumps.

4 Pour boiling broth into pan, standing back (it will spatter) as you do so.

5 Lower heat, cover pan, and simmer for approximately 20 minutes, or until broth is absorbed and kasha is fluffy.

6 In saucepan, sauté giblets, onions, and garlic until soft. Add to kasha, then add wine and pecans. Mix well, making sure mixture is well moistened.

7 The dressing will dry out if exposed to oven heat. If you bake it in a casserole, cover pan with foil to prevent drying out.

8 Bake for 30 minutes, or until heated through.

Makes 4–6 servings

GF Bread Dressing

5–6 cups GF English muffins,
　　buns, or bread, cut into
　　2" cubes
2 tablespoons oil
3 cups celery, chopped
2 cups onion, chopped
1 teaspoon thyme
1 teaspoon parsley
1 teaspoon salt
Black pepper
1½ cups GF broth

Everyone has a favorite turkey dressing recipe. This recipe appeared in the Miss Robens (now known as Allergy Grocer) catalog; I modified it a little to suit my family's taste. I found that using GF English muffins worked especially well because they are thick enough to cut into cubes. I used the muffins made by Foods by George, a GF bakery in New Jersey. Other English muffins would work too, as would GF bread.

According to my mother, a loose rule of thumb says about 10 cups bread pieces makes enough for a 10-pound bird.

1 Preheat oven to 325°F.

2 Spread English muffin cubes on a cookie sheet.

3 Toast cubes for 30 minutes or so. Shake pan or turn with a spatula every 10 minutes. Cubes should be well dried. They do not need to be browned, but it is fine if they are.

4 Sauté celery and onion in oil over medium heat until soft. Add herbs and spices.

5 Pour in broth and simmer over low heat for 15–20 minutes.

6 Add muffin cubes to saucepan, and combine until cubes are fully saturated in sauce and seasonings.

7 Transfer to a covered casserole dish and change oven temperature to 400°F.

8 Bake casserole for 40–50 minutes.

Makes 4–6 servings

Cranberry Nut Dressing

I adore cranberries. Every November, when they first make their appearance in the grocery store, I buy enough to last the year. They freeze very well, and I love to throw them into applesauce and other dishes. I also like dried cranberries, which used to be hard to find but now are widely available. This recipe uses dried cranberries and nuts, and is a really nice change of pace.

1 Preheat oven to 325°F.
2 Sauté celery and onion in margarine, and remove from heat when tender. Add herbs, salt, and pepper.
3 Place bread cubes in a mixing bowl, and add celery mixture, cranberries, and nuts. Use enough broth to moisten well.
4 Bake mixture in a covered casserole for 30–45 minutes.

Makes 4–6 servings

½ cup celery, chopped
½ cup onion, chopped
¼ cup CF margarine
½ teaspoon dried thyme
½ teaspoon dried marjoram
Salt and pepper (to taste)
6 cups bread (preferably GF
   English Muffins), cubed
   and toasted lightly
½ cup dried cranberries
½ cup nuts, chopped
   (preferably pecans
   or hazelnuts)
½ cup GF chicken broth

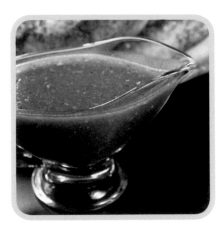

Gravy

There's no mystery to making GF gravy. If you are grain-free, you can cook the giblets in broth until it is reduced enough to thicken a little (it will not be thick). If you can use appropriate flours, you can make it the traditional way.

1 While turkey is roasting, bring stock to a boil in a medium saucepan.

2 Add giblets and neck, then lower heat.

3 Simmer giblets for about 1 hour, until it reduces to 4 cups.

4 Add 2–4 tablespoons of roasting pan fat to mixture, and cook on high heat until reduced to 2 cups.

5 Remove giblets and neck, and pour ½ cup liquid into a small bowl. Add cornstarch to liquid, and stir until well dissolved.

6 Add liquid back to pan and cook over low heat, stirring often, until gravy has thickened.

Makes 4–6 servings

Turkey giblets and neck

6 cups chicken stock

2–4 tablespoons fat from
    roasting pan of turkey

3 tablespoons cornstarch*

 If your child cannot eat corn products, sweet rice flour or tapioca starch flour may be substituted.

Roast Goose

Geese and ducks are served less commonly than turkey, even though they are tasty and easy to make. Geese, like all water fowl, need a lot of fat to keep warm. This means they are very delicious, but it also means that you do not get a lot of flesh from even a large bird. In fact, by the time the fat has melted away, you probably need to allow for 1 pound per person. Really large geese are not that easy to find, so you may need to buy more than one small bird if you are feeding a crowd of more than eight. You can use any dressing you would use for turkey, or you can skip it altogether.

1 (8-pound) goose
Large orange (optional)
Salt and pepper (to taste)
12 bacon slices (nitrite free), divided
2 tablespoons GF breadcrumbs
¼ cup fresh herbs, minced (e.g., parsley, basil, thyme)
1 tablespoon Dijon mustard

1 Preheat oven to 425°F.

2 Remove giblets and set aside for making dressing (see recipes for GF Bread Dressing on page 246). Pierce skin of bird with a fork.

3 If you stuff goose, fill body and neck cavity with stuffing. If you choose not to stuff goose, place orange in body cavity.

4 Place bird on a meat rack in a roasting pan. Cover bird with bacon; set aside remaining bacon. Roast goose for 45 minutes, pouring off fat as needed.

5 Reduce oven heat to 375°F and bake for another 60–90 minutes (longer if the bird is stuffed).

6 Chop remaining bacon very finely and mix with herbs and bread crumbs.

7 Spread mustard on goose and cover with bread crumbs and bake another 20–30 minutes, or until meat is tender and juice runs clear.

Makes 8 servings

Stuffed Pork Tenderloin

½ cup onion, chopped
½ cup celery, chopped
1½ cups chicken broth
6 cups GF English muffins,
    cubed and dry
½ teaspoon dried thyme
1 teaspoon dried marjoram
1 teaspoon dried parsley
1 (1½-pound) pork tenderloin
½ teaspoon salt
1 teaspoon pepper

This recipe is delicious, and is deceptively easy (i.e., it will look as though you really fussed). If you are not feeding a large crowd, this can make a nice main course. Any stuffing recipe would work with this recipe. As usual, I have omitted the sage, but if you like it, use ½ teaspoon. **Note**: Cube the English muffins and leave them out to dry for a day. If you do not remember to do this, just put them on a cookie sheet and toast in a 325°F oven for 30 minutes or so, until well dried out. If you have leftover stuffing, skip to the part of the recipe when pork is sliced.

1 Preheat oven to 350°F.
2 In a large saucepan, combine onion, celery, and broth. Simmer, covered, on low until vegetables are soft.
3 Remove from heat and add bread and herbs, and mix until blended. Set aside stuffing.
4 Slice pork into ¼" slices.
5 Arrange half the slices in a baking pan that has been sprayed with non-stick cooking spray. Top with stuffing. Place remaining pork slices on stuffing. Sprinkle with salt and pepper. Cover with aluminum foil.
6 Bake for 30 minutes, or until pork is no longer pink.

Makes 4–6 servings

Roast Leg of Lamb

If your family likes lamb, roasting a leg of lamb is another great choice for the holidays. My husband's family is French, and it was at my mother-in-law's table that I first had a fabulous "gigot" smothered in garlic and cooked deliciously rare. Served with small potatoes, or just about anything you want, this will be a wonderful centerpiece for your meal, and will not cost you hours of hard labor in the kitchen. In France leg of lamb is often accompanied by flageolet, which are tiny greenish-white beans. They can be hard to find, but are available online from many bean companies such as www.purcellmountainfarms.com.

Note: Many stores are now carrying boned, butterflied leg of lamb. They seem more expensive, but there is no waste, and they cook quickly in the oven or on the grill.

1 Preheat oven to 350°F.

2 Trim excess fat from lamb, and season with salt and pepper.

3 Combine mustard, juice, garlic, onion, and herbs in a blender. Blend to emulsify. Slowly trickle in oil.

4 At least 1 hour before roasting, baste lamb with mustard mixture, and set it on a rack in a heavy-duty roasting pan.

5 Roast lamb for 1–1¼ hours for medium rare (140°F–145F° on meat thermometer). Roast lamb for 1¼–1½ hours for well-done meat (160°F–165°F on meat thermometer).

6 Remove lamb from roasting pan and place on a warm platter. Let lamb rest for 15 minutes before carving.

7 Pour off pan drippings and remove as much fat as possible. Season to taste and serve drippings with meat.

Makes 4–6 servings

1 (6-pound) leg of lamb, bone in
Kosher or coarse salt (to taste)
Pepper (to taste)
¼ cup Dijon mustard
2 tablespoons lemon juice
4 fresh garlic cloves, minced
1 large onion, peeled and chopped
1 tablespoon fresh rosemary, finely chopped
1 tablespoon fresh thyme, finely chopped
1 tablespoon fresh mint, finely chopped
2 tablespoons extra virgin olive oil

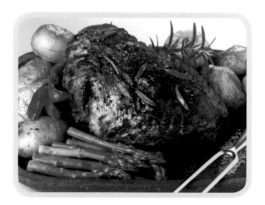

✳ Baked Cranberry Sauce

⅓ cup sugar

1 (6-ounce) jar orange marmalade

½ cup pecans, chopped (optional)

1 (12-ounce) package cranberries

1 cup dried cherries (or berries) (optional)

The recipe on the back of the Ocean Spray package is easy to make and very good, but I often add other ingredients, usually dried cherries. A few years ago I found this recipe, and I love the ease of putting it in the oven (no stirring a pot of messy, popping berries). This recipe is convenient, especially when you have lots of other things to cook. Cooled, covered cranberries hold well in the fridge, so you can make it a day or two ahead to save time.

1 Preheat oven to 350°F.

2 Lightly grease an 8" pan, or spray with cooking spray.

3 In a medium bowl, mix sugar, marmalade, and nuts. Then stir in cranberries and dried fruit.

4 Pour mixture into pan and bake for 35–40 minutes.

5 Serve warm.

Makes 4–6 servings

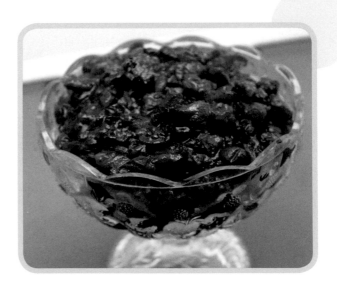

Root-Vegetable Mashed Potatoes with Chestnuts

This dish makes a nice change of pace from plain mashed potatoes. The parsnips are usually tolerated, even by children with food sensitivities, and they add some extra nutrients and fiber. Chestnuts are also well tolerated, and are the only nut that is truly low in fat.

1 Place potatoes, parsnips, and garlic in a large saucepan.

2 Cover with water and bring to a boil.

3 Cook vegetables for 20 minutes or until very tender. Drain.

4 Return potato mixture to pan, then add broth, margarine, and parsley.

5 Using a hand mixer set at medium speed, beat until smooth.

6 Stir in chestnuts and seasonings.

Makes 4–6 servings

4 cups potatoes, peeled
    and cubed (Yukon Gold
    work well)
2 cups parsnips, peeled
    and sliced
5 garlic cloves, peeled
Water
¼ cup GF chicken broth
1 tablespoon CF margarine
¼ cup fresh parsley, chopped
½ cup chestnuts, cooked,
    shelled, and chopped
Salt and pepper (to taste)

Mashed Sweet Potatoes

4 sweet potatoes, roasted and
   peeled
6 tablespoons CF margarine
½ cup Darifree™, warmed
   (or soy milk)
1 egg, lightly beaten
½ teaspoon nutmeg (optional)
Salt and pepper (to taste)

Sweet potatoes do not have to be made dessert-sweet.
Mash them instead of regular russet potatoes for a nice
holiday starch.

1 Preheat oven to 350°F.
2 In a large bowl, mash sweet potatoes with margarine.
3 Beat in milk substitute, egg, and spices.
4 Transfer to a lightly greased casserole and bake for
25 minutes.
5 Serve hot.

Makes 4–6 servings

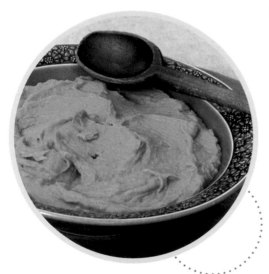

✻ Mashed Christmas Beans

After reading Barbara Kingsolver's wonderful book, *Animal, Vegetable, Miracle*, I was inspired to get more beans into our diet. She talked about mashing colorful Christmas lima beans, and I had to try it. These are really mild, nutty tasting beans, and they make a wonderful holiday side dish that is really different. Even non-bean eaters will like this! You can buy the beans from Purcellmountainfarms.com if you do not find them locally.

1 (1–pound) package
    Christmas lima beans
Water
Vegetable broth

1 Wash and pick over beans, removing any debris.
2 Cover with cold water and soak for 3 hours or overnight at room temperature.
3 Drain water and rinse well, then cover with 2" fresh water.
4 Bring beans to a simmer and cook gently for 1–2 hours, until very tender.
5 Mash or puree the beans, adding a little vegetable broth if needed to get desired texture.

Makes 4–6 servings

Roasted Vegetables

Potatoes (one or
  more varieties)
Parsnips
Sweet potatoes
Carrots
Onions
Any other root vegetable
Olive oil (or other oil)
Salt and pepper (to taste)

When the holiday table is groaning with heavy dishes and lots of artery-clogging goodies, it is nice to include something light and virtuous. A few years ago my mother started serving roasted veggies with her holiday meals, and I have taken a page from her book. Even if your children are not big veggie eaters, they will probably accept the potatoes. Adjust the amounts to the number of people at your table, and do not save these just for holidays. You can also make these on the grill for a great addition to any picnic.

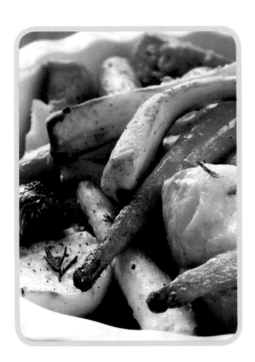

1 Preheat oven to 425°F.
2 Cut vegetables into large chunks.
3 Spread out vegetables on a cookie sheet that has been lightly sprayed with cooking oil. (I usually line the pan with non-stick foil first.)
4 Drizzle with oil, and season with salt and pepper.
5 Roast vegetables in oven for 40 minutes.
6 Decrease oven temperature to 375°F, and roast for another 20 minutes.
7 Serve hot or warm.

Servings will vary.

Gingerbread People

What could be sweeter than little gingerbread folk? I usually make mine in a variety of sizes, and often stick a small cookie hand on the hand of the large Mommy cookie. I even have a tiny boy and girl cookie cutter — these get pressed across the front of the Mommy cookie, and her arms are folded around the baby. Little girl cookies hold the tiny ones as dolls, and little boy cookies are baked, perched upon the Dad cookie's shoulders. It may be hard to picture, but when decorated with royal icing, they are quite lovely. This recipe comes by way of Karyn Seroussi. I have also used recipes adapted from old favorites.

1 Preheat oven to 350°F.
2 Combine dry ingredients in a large bowl. Then add oil, molasses, and water.
3 Mix well, adding more tapioca starch flour as needed to make a soft dough that can be kneaded.
4 Roll out dough on a tapioca-floured board to a thickness of ¼".
5 Cut out dough with gingerbread-people cutters, dipping cutters into tapioca starch flour after each use.
6 Bake cookies on ungreased cookie sheets for approximately 14 minutes.
7 Remove cookies from pan while hot; cool on a wire rack. Cookies will be slightly chewy.

Makes 36 cookies

⅔ cup brown rice flour
⅓ cup sweet rice flour
⅓ cup tapioca starch flour
¼ cup sugar
I tablespoon cinnamon
2 teaspoons xanthan gum
I teaspoon ginger (to taste)
I teaspoon GF baking soda
½ teaspoon salt
¼ cup oil
¼ cup molasses
2 tablespoons water
Royal icing*

*Royal icing is generally used on gingerbread people; it is also the "mortar" that holds gingerbread houses together. It is basically sugar, egg whites, and water   not exactly a health food, but it is used in small amounts for special occasions. I buy a meringue powder mix from www. kingarthurflour.com when I need royal icing. Or I use Wilton icing mix, which is available at cake decorating stores and party stores, as well as some groceries.

Spritz Cookies

¾ cup sugar

1 cup CF margarine, at room
    temperature

1 egg

1 teaspoon pure almond
    extract

1 teaspoon vanilla flavoring

2 cups GF flour mix

½ cup almond flour*

Pinch salt (optional)

 *Almond flour is just finely
ground almonds. If you
cannot find it, you can
make your own in a blender or food
processor. Take care — if you go too
far it will be almond butter. It is usually available in health food stores,
and there are many online sources too.

My maternal grandmother, Bubby Mary, was a wonderful baker. Much of what I know about baking I learned from her. My mother often dropped me off to spend an afternoon with Bubby, and we always baked something together. She loved to make Spritz cookies, and always used a cookie press to make them look fancy. Without gluten, however, the dough is too soft to put through a cookie press. Instead, I use a pastry bag filled with a large star tip (#6). Pastry bags and tips are sold in stores that carry cake decorating supplies, and in the baking section of most supermarkets. These are perfect for Christmastime, and always find their way into the gift baskets I prepare.

1 Preheat oven to 375°F.

2 Using an electric mixer, cream together sugar and margarine until fluffy. Add egg and flavorings; beat until well blended.

3 On low speed, gradually add flours and salt. Mix until incorporated.

4 Place dough in pastry bag (already fitted with star tip), and fill about halfway.** (If you overfill your pastry bag, dough will squirt out the top, making a real mess.)

5 Line baking sheets with parchment, and hold pastry bag at a 90° angle from sheet. Squeeze out desired amount of dough to make a star shape, or lower the angle of the bag slightly and move in a circular direction to make a rosette. Make cookies about 1¾" in diameter.

6 For the best shape, hold tip very close to, but not touching, baking sheet. Squeeze firmly until cookie is the size you want, and then lift tip straight up to finish.

7 Decorate cookies with whatever you would like. You could use glace cherries and other fruits, pearl sugar, sprinkles (use in moderation due to the artificial colors and starches), coconut, or even GFCF chocolate chips. Granulated sugar can be colored with a few drops of concentrated fruit juice, or you can buy naturally colored sugar online (e.g., www.naturesflavors.com, http://organic.lovetoknow.com/Natural_Food_Coloring). Note that if you color your own sugar, it must be done in advance to allow time for drying.

8 Bake in center of oven for 10–12 minutes. Rotate sheet midway through baking, and if you are using two sheets at once, rotate and exchange top to bottom as well.

9 Cool on racks and store in airtight containers. Cooled cookies freeze well if wrapped tightly.

Makes 36 cookies

**If you have never used a pastry bag before, I suggest buying a set of disposable bags and tips (usually available with cake mixes and icings in the grocery store). Then watch one of the many Youtube videos on "how to use a pastry bag."

✳ Refrigerator Pumpkin Pie

A few years ago, I became fascinated with the old-fashioned concept of the "icebox" pie. What attracted me about these pies is that they have a cracker- or cookie-crumb crust, which is particularly easy to modify for my son's dietary restrictions. In addition, they must be made ahead of time, so it is one less thing to worry about when busily preparing a big holiday meal. A few years ago, I made a pumpkin pie for Thanksgiving, using Mi-Del GF Ginger Snaps (available in many big stores and in health food stores) for the crust. Everyone loved this pie, and now I make it every year. **Note:** This mousse pie calls for whipped cream, which obviously will not work if you are avoiding dairy. There are whipped cream substitutes available, but they are filled with high fructose corn syrup, soy products, and a ton of sugar. Instead, try making it with whipped cashew cream or coconut whipped "cream" (see recipe on page 347).

This pie will need to chill for at least 8 hours, so it is not a "last-minute" recipe! If you really want to get a jump on the holidays, you can make this crust up to a month ahead, and freeze it tightly wrapped. It is a great time saver if you have the freezer space.

Ginger Snap Crust

20–30 GF ginger snap cookies
5 tablespoons CF margarine, melted and cooled
½ teaspoon ground cinnamon
⅛ teaspoon salt

1 Preheat oven to 350°F.
2 Put cookies in food processor or blender and process until finely ground.
3 Measure 1 ⅓ cups of cookie crumbs. Transfer to a medium bowl, and add remaining ingredients.
4 Mix until crumbs are evenly moist. The texture will be like damp sand.

5 Press crumb mixture into bottom and up sides of a 9″ pie pan. Pack it in as evenly and tightly as you can. (I have a tiny rolling pin for this, but the bottom and side of a small glass will also work to press the crumbs up the side nicely.)

6 Bake crust until crisp and lightly browned, about 8 minutes.

7 Cool completely before filling.

Makes I (9-inch) pie crust

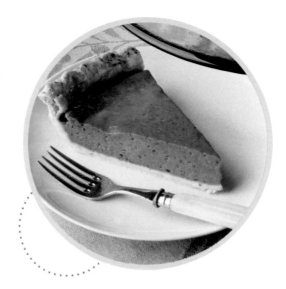

Pumpkin Filling

I Put I tablespoon cold water in a small stainless steel bowl, and sprinkle gelatin on top. Let stand until gelatin dissolves.

2 Put a few inches water in bottom of a double boiler, and bring it to a simmer (not a rolling boil). In top of double boiler, whisk together egg yolks and sugar. Whisk constantly until egg mixture reaches 160°F on an instant-read thermometer.

3 Remove pan from heat, and whisk in gelatin-water mixture. Beat this with an electric mixer until it is cool and thick for about 5 minutes. Beat in pumpkin and spices.

4 Gently fold coconut cream (reserving a few spoonfuls) into pumpkin mixture, then scrape into cooled crust.

5 Cover pie with plastic wrap, and chill for at least 8 hours, until completely set.

6 Serve with dollops of reserved coconut cream.

Makes I (9-inch) pie

Water

I teaspoon unflavored gelatin

3 egg yolks

½ cup sugar

I cup unsweetened pumpkin purée

½ teaspoon ground ginger

¼ teaspoon ground cloves

¼ teaspoon ground nutmeg

I cup coconut whipped "cream" (see recipe on page 347)

Pie crust (see Ginger Snap Crust recipe on page 260)

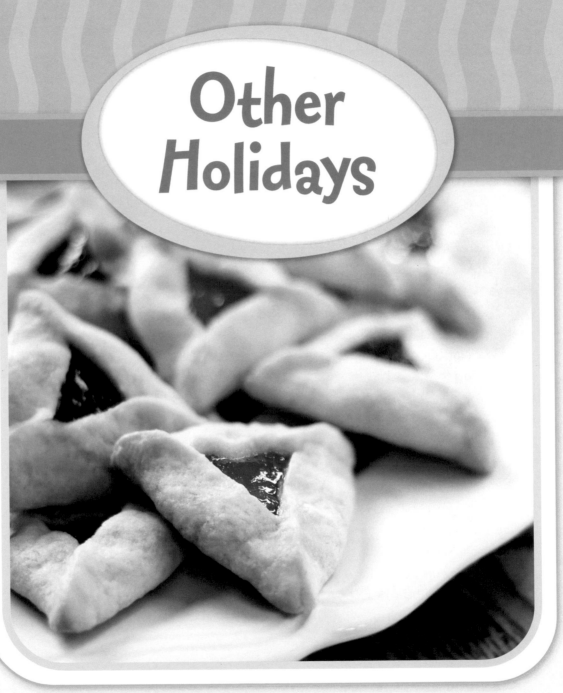

Other Holidays

Hamentashen, recipe on page 269

Potato Pancakes (Latkes)

Often served on Hanukkah, potato latkes are delicious with chicken or meat. Like large Tater Tots, only better, they are too good to make only once a year. Most grocery stores stock potato pancake mixes in the Kosher section. They taste fairly good, but unfortunately nearly all brands add sulfites to the potatoes, so read labels carefully. Since sulfites are intended to keep the potato white, it is a little silly — latkes are brown when cooked anyway! With today's food processors, it is a snap to grate potatoes and make these from scratch.

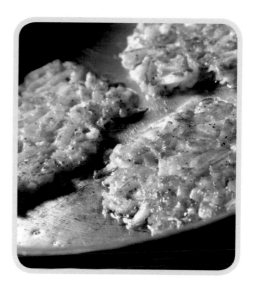

1 Peel and grate potatoes. Squeeze out as much liquid as possible from potatoes.
2 Add eggs, salt, and enough crumbs so mixture is stiff enough to form into patties.
3 Heat oil in a frying pan for a few minutes.
4 Use crumb mixture to form latkes with wet hands.
5 Fry latkes until golden and crispy on all sides.

Servings will vary.

3 potatoes, peeled
2 eggs
Pinch Salt
¼ cup GF bread crumbs
Oil

Matzo Balls (Kneidlach)

½ cup roasted baby
    rice cereal
    (with no fillers)
1 egg
1 tablespoon oil
½ teaspoon GF baking
    powder
Pinch salt

Matzo balls are light, airy dumplings made, traditionally, at Passover. They are always served floating in a flavorful chicken soup. Matzo, however, is made from wheat flour. I could not bear the thought of a Passover Seder with no matzo balls, and was complaining about it to my mother. She remembered that years ago, some women had made their matzo balls from Cream of Wheat cereal. I had never heard of that before, but tried it, using rice cereal. After a few trials, I determined that the roasted baby rice cereal found at the health food store made the best matzo balls. A tradition was born (or reborn).

Then, a couple of years ago, I found something that made even better matzo balls! "Pesach Crumbs" are made from egg white and potato starch, and for some reason they make terrific matzo balls. They are only available for a limited time, around Passover (in the spring). Some stores that have big Kosher sections carry it, or check with www.mykoshermarket.com about 6 weeks before Passover. The crumbs also make an excellent breading substitute. When I find Pesach Crumbs, I buy enough to last the year and store them in the freezer. (They will go rancid if left on a shelf for more than a few weeks.)

1 Mix all ingredients in a bowl, combining well.
2 Cover bowl with plastic wrap and let rest in refrigerator for at least 20 minutes.
3 Bring a large pot of water to a boil.
4 With wet or oiled hands, form chilled mixture in small balls, and drop them into boiling water. (Matzo balls expand to several times their original size — do not make balls larger than walnuts, or you will have grapefruit-sized matzo balls!)
5 Boil matzo balls, covered, for 30–40 minutes. When done, balls will float to top of pot.
6 Remove cooked matzo balls with a slotted spoon.
7 Place 1–3 matzo balls in each bowl, and serve in homemade soup.

Makes 4–6 servings

Bean Flour Matzo

Passover matzo is always made from wheat, and I am often asked how to make it from other flours. I usually skip it, but one year Sam's teacher asked me to send in some matzo that Sam could eat. This recipe was originally a Bette Hagman pasta recipe, then was modified by Gina Levy and posted to the Yahoo group Gfcfrecipes (http://health.groups.yahoo.com/group/GFCFrecipes/. Now there are GF matzos available commercially, but they cost a fortune (almost $20 a box!) and, the one time I splurged, they were nearly all broken and crumbly.

⅓ cup tapioca starch flour
⅓ cup cornstarch, plus additional for kneading (or potato starch)
⅓ cup Garfava Flour
2 teaspoons xanthan gum
½ teaspoon salt (optional)
2 eggs
1 tablespoon olive oil

1 Preheat oven to 400°F.
2 In a medium bowl, combine starches, flour, salt, and xanthan gum.
3 Whisk together eggs and oil, pour into dry ingredients, and stir until a ball forms.
4 Knead mixture for 1–2 minutes, adding more cornstarch if necessary. Work in cornstarch until dough will not accept any more, and is firm.
5 Place ball of dough on a cutting board dusted with cornstarch, and roll as thin as possible.
6 Cut dough into matzo-board shapes, and poke rows of holes with a fork.
7 Carefully lift matzo onto an ungreased cookie sheet.
8 Bake matzo for 8–10 minutes, or until crispy.

Makes 4–6 servings

Passover Rolls

1½ cups water
¼ cup safflower oil
½ teaspoon salt
2¼ cups Pesach Crumbs
4 eggs

These rolls are typically made with matzo meal during the Jewish holiday of Passover. Since matzo meal contains gluten, try making them with Paskesz Pesach Crumbs. These "crumbs" are made from potato starch and egg, and can be used for any recipe that calls for matzo meal. They are available only during the Passover season, so when spring comes, try finding them in a Kosher market. Or visit a website such as www.mykoshermarket.com. You can also try www.kosher.com. **Note:** Both online stores close several days before Passover, so shop early. If you cannot get Pesach Crumbs, try substituting ground Hol Grain crackers or Schär brand GF cracker crumbs.

1 Preheat oven to 375°F.
2 Bring water, oil, and salt to a boil in a medium saucepan over medium-low heat.
3 Remove from heat and add crumbs. Mix well.
4 Return pan to low heat and cook, stirring for 1 minute. Remove from heat and cool 5 minutes.
5 Place crumb mixture in a mixer fitted with flat paddle; beat in 1 egg.
6 When mixture is smooth, beat in another egg. Continue adding eggs one by one, beating after each addition.
7 Drop 2 tablespoons batter, for each roll, onto parchment–lined baking sheets. Allow about 1½" between rolls.
8 Bake rolls for about 30–40 minutes, or until golden brown and firm.

Makes 18 rolls

Mandel Bread

Mandel Bread (or Kamish Broit) is basically Jewish biscotti! It is a twice-baked cookie that is very crispy (and dunkable, if you are so inclined). My mother and her mother always made these cookies for Hanukkah. Their recipe adapted very easily to GF flour, so they are again a Hanukkah staple for us. For fancier cookies, divide the dough into four pieces. The resulting cookies will be much smaller and will look nicer.

1 Preheat oven to 350°F.

2 Beat eggs, oil, and sugar in a bowl. Add baking powder, flour, xanthan gum, salt, and vanilla (it will be a stiff batter).

3 Shape batter into 2 thin loaves on a greased cookie sheet.

4 Bake 30 minutes until light brown.

5 Slice loaves on diagonal while still warm. Lay slices on cut side, sprinkle with cinnamon and sugar mixture.

6 Decrease oven temperature to 300°F, and toast loaves until crispy and brown, for about 45 minutes.

Makes 2 small loaves

6 eggs
½ cup oil
I cup sugar
I teaspoon GF baking powder
3 cups GF flour
2 teaspoons xanthan gum
I teaspoon salt
I teaspoon pure vanilla extract
Cinnamon and sugar mixture

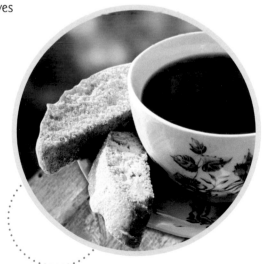

✴ *new* Mandel Bread II

1 stick CF margarine, softened

1½ cups sugar

2 teaspoons pure vanilla
    extract

4 eggs

2 cups GF flour blend

2 teaspoons xanthan gum

1 teaspoon cinnamon

½ teaspoon GF baking powder

2 cups nuts, chopped
    (almonds, walnuts, or
    pecans)

Cinnamon and sugar mixture
    (optional)

I was served this mandel bread at my mother's home, and I could not get over how good it was. If your family likes a crunchy cookie, this will be a real winner. This cookie is twice baked but unlike the previous recipe, it must be frozen before the second baking. It is nice to keep some of these in the freezer because it takes little time to complete them for freshly baked cookies.

1 Preheat oven to 350°F.

2 Cream margarine with sugar in a bowl. Add vanilla and then eggs, one at a time.

3 Combine dry ingredients (except nuts and cinnamon sugar mixture), and then add them to liquid mixture. Add nuts.

4 Divide batter between 3 greased 5"x 2½"x 2" (mini loaf) pans.

5 Bake loaves for 30 minutes.

6 Cool completely. Wrap in foil and freeze.

7 When ready to serve, thaw loaves for about 15 minutes, slice thinly, and sprinkle with cinnamon sugar mixture.

8 Lower oven heat to 300°F and bake for 10 minutes on each side (they will look like Melba toast when ready).

Makes 3 small loaves

Hamentashen

This is a treat served for the Jewish holiday of Purim. They have become very popular, however, and are often available year-round in bakeries and stores on the East Coast. The cookies are soft (unless you overbake), and they freeze well. If made small, they look nice enough for a fancy tray.

1 Preheat oven to 350°F.

2 Cream sugar and oil, then add eggs and blend well. Stir in vanilla.

3 Mix together dry ingredients, and add to liquid mixture.

4 Roll out dough on a GF-floured surface.

5 Cut dough into 2½" circles.

6 Place 1 teaspoon filling on each cookie, and moisten edges of dough with water.

7 Bring together sides of cookie to form a triangle, with the filling peeking through middle. Pinch edges of dough to hold shape.

8 Bake cookies on a lightly greased sheet for 10–15 minutes.

Makes 36 cookies

1½ cups sugar

1 cup vegetable oil

4 eggs

1 teaspoon pure vanilla extract

4½ cups GF flour

4 teaspoons GF baking powder

2 teaspoons xanthan gum

¼ teaspoon salt

1 (15-ounce) can cherry pie filling (or apricot fruit jam)*

 *Most stores carry various brands. Check ingredients carefully, since many of these fillings contain starch. Most use tapioca, which is fine, but make sure the label states the source of starch.

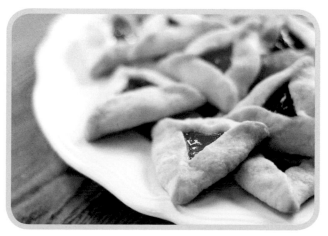

Ethnic Foods

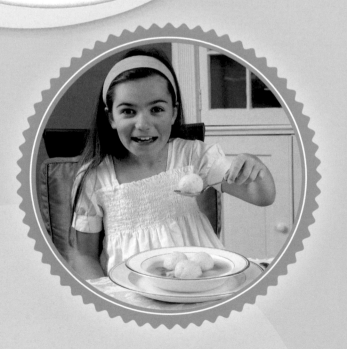

The typical American diet is very wheat- and dairy-centric, which is why it is often so hard to make dietary changes and stick to them. This is not true of every cuisine, however, so I always advise newbies to head out to the library and check out cookbooks featuring non-American foods. Most libraries have large cookbook collections and borrowing them is an inexpensive way to broaden your cooking horizons. Sometimes there will only be one or two recipes that interest you, and for a few quarters you can copy those pages right in the library. Do not assume that your family will not eat "foreign" food—all food is foreign until you are introduced to it. Here are a few favorites to get you started before you head out to the library!

Chicken Soup

1 stewing chicken
(use the largest you can fit
in your pot)

Water

2 teaspoons salt

1 onion, chopped

1 garlic clove, minced

2 large carrots, peeled and
chopped

1 parsnip, peeled

2 celery stalks, strings removed
and chopped

2–3 fresh parsley sprigs

Pepper (to taste)

1 quart GF canned chicken
broth (optional)

 Note: *When my mother wants an especially wonderful soup, she makes what she calls Double Chicken Soup. For this soup, she makes the chicken soup and strains it carefully. She then uses the broth (instead of water) to cook a second chicken, prepared as above. Soup prepared this way is so rich it is nearly brown, and is particularly flavorful.*

In addition to being good for cold and flu sufferers, chicken soup is delicious. Served with GF noodles or matzo balls (see chapter 9), it is a wonderful way to start a meal. I also love chicken soup with cooked kasha (buckwheat groats). The vegetables in the soup add flavor and nutrition, but by the time the flavor has been cooked into the soup, they are quite mushy. Many soups and casseroles call for broth, and none is as good as homemade. To have chicken broth on hand, strain it well and let it come to room temperature. Remove any fat that rises to the top, then freeze in appropriate containers.

1 Rinse chicken thoroughly, then place in a large pot and cover with water. Add salt and bring to a boil. (Be sure to include the giblets.)

2 Let chicken cook for about 20 minutes on low heat, skimming the foam off the surface of the water as it collects. When very little foam is collecting on the surface, add remaining ingredients to the pot (except carrots and celery).

3 Lower the heat and simmer the soup for approximately 2½ hours, checking occasionally to make sure there is enough liquid. If needed, add water or canned chicken broth.

4 Taste and correct seasonings, then strain the broth carefully and return the clear soup to the pot.

5 Return some of the cooked chicken to the soup, if desired, and increase the volume by adding more canned broth if necessary. Add carrot and celery and cook for another 30 minutes, until the vegetables are tender but not mushy.

6 Refrigerate the soup until fat congeals on top. Skim off fat with a spoon.

7 Reheat soup before serving. Matzo balls, GF noodles, or kasha may be served in the soup, but should be cooked separately. Place these in the bowl, then ladle soup to cover.

Makes 4 servings

Variation: For a child who is extremely reactive to foods and pigments, a white version of the soup can be made by omitting the carrots and parsley and adding 4 stalks bok choy cabbage (white part only).

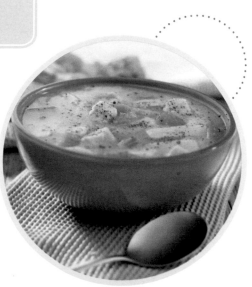

Unchicken Soup

8 quarts water

2 teaspoons salt

2 onions, chopped

2 garlic cloves, minced

2 parsnips, peeled

8 bok choy cabbage stalks,
    white part only

4–6 fresh parsley sprigs

Pepper (to taste)

4 large carrots, peeled and
    chopped

4 celery stalks, strings removed
    and chopped

¼–½ teaspoon turmeric

For people who cannot eat chicken, or who are vegetarians, you can make a version of this soup without the chicken. It is very tasty, and like the soups made with chicken, leftover broth adds flavor and nutrition when cooking rice and other grains.

1 To make this soup, bring water to boil in a large pot. Add remaining ingredients (except carrots, celery, and turmeric).

2 Cook on low heat until broth has taken on color and flavor of ingredients. Vegetables should be very soft.

3 Strain broth and return it to pot.

4 Correct seasonings, and add carrot and celery. Cook gently until carrot and celery pieces are soft, but not mushy.

5 Remove from heat and stir in turmeric, which gives the soup a yellow coloring.

6 This soup freezes well.

Makes 4 servings

Mock Chopped Liver

This is a strange recipe. It contains no meat, yet really tastes like traditional Jewish chopped liver. It makes a nice appetizer for the grown-ups who are watching their cholesterol and would never dream of eating the real thing. If your children eat it too, that is great. I have seen versions of this recipe in lots of magazines — this is one I got from my mother, who has no idea where she got it.

2 onions, chopped
Oil
5 hard-boiled eggs, whites only
I cup chopped walnuts
I (8-ounce) can of peas,
　drained but reserve liquid
Salt and pepper (to taste)

I Sauté onions in oil until very brown.
2 Place onions, egg whites, walnuts, and peas in a food processor or blender, using most of the liquid from the peas. If it seems dry, add the rest of the liquid.
3 Season with salt and pepper, and chill thoroughly.

Makes 4 servings

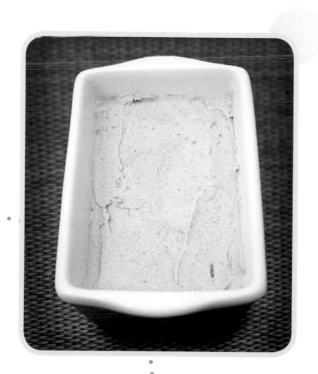

Ozzie's Mock Chopped Liver

¾ cup lentils
3 cups chicken broth
1 very large onion
    (or 2 medium onions)
Oil
2 hard-boiled eggs, whites only
Salt and pepper (to taste)

A few years ago, I was asked to teach a class at a New York cooking school. They wanted me to talk about how to make GFCF holiday food, and the cooking students provided some wonderful food for everyone to sample. One of the treats was a mock chopped liver made of lentils — it was absolutely delicious. I really wanted the recipe, but the person who had made it did not stay for the class. Then last December my mother's friend, Ozzie Nogg, brought the same thing to a gathering at my parents' home. I was so happy to find it again, and to finally have the recipe! It is a really good appetizer, nutritious and tasty.

1 Cook lentils in broth, simmering for about 35 minutes. Cover and simmer until tender.
2 Sauté onion in oil until well caramelized.
3 Drain lentils, reserving some liquid.
4 Put all ingredients in a food processor and process well. If too dry, add a touch of reserved liquid.
5 Season to taste and serve with GF crackers.

Makes 4 servings

Falafel

Falafel is sold everywhere in Israel, but especially in the Arab market, where falafel wagons are as common as hot dog vendors in New York. On the streets, falafels are usually stuffed into pita bread, sandwich-style, and covered with enough hot sauce to make you go back and buy that (expensive) imported soda. In Middle Eastern restaurants in the United States, they are generally served on a plate, with pita or flatbread on the side. Add some hummus or baba ghanoush, and you have a wonderful Middle Eastern meal. If you do not have time to make it yourself, there are excellent frozen falafel available at Whole Foods and other special markets.

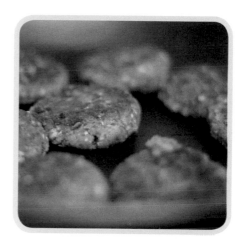

1 Process chickpeas and water in a blender or food processor until smooth. Add remaining ingredients (except flour and oil) and blend well.

2 Add just enough GF flour to the mixture to form a dough. With wet hands, form dough into small balls, the size of a large walnut.

3 Fry falafel in a pot with oil, until brown and crispy on all sides. Keep falafel moving in the pot, or they will stick. (They sink at first!)

4 Remove to a paper towel-lined plate and blot excess oil with additional paper towels.

5 Serve immediately with flatbread (e.g., tortillas, Chapatis) and tahini sauce, which has been thinned with lemon juice and hot sauce.

Makes 4 servings

2 cups chickpeas, cooked
  (drain and rinse well if using
  canned beans)
½ cup water
1 onion, chopped
1–2 garlic cloves, minced or
  put through a garlic press
1 fresh parsley sprig, minced
1 tablespoon cumin
1½ teaspoons coriander
1 teaspoon cayenne pepper
  (less for milder falafel)
1 teaspoon salt
½ cup soy or other heavy
  GF flour (e.g., brown rice,
  Jowar, quinoa)
½ cup oil

Baba Ghanoush

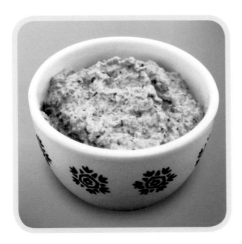

Even people who swear they do not like eggplant enjoy this dish. It can be used as a sandwich spread or a dip. It is best scooped up and eaten with a flatbread.

1 medium eggplant
2 garlic cloves (more if desired)
¼ cup freshly squeezed
    lemon juice
¼ cup tahini
    (available at most groceries
    and health food stores)
Salt and pepper (to taste)

1 Preheat oven to 350°F.
2 Lightly grease outside of eggplant, and bake on a sprayed cookie sheet until very tender, around 30 minutes, depending on the size of eggplant. It is OK if the outside of eggplant chars a little, but be sure to turn it several times during baking.
3 When eggplant has cooled, cut it in half and scoop out the inside.
4 Add remaining ingredients to eggplant and puree in a food processor or blender. I usually put all the ingredients in a bowl and use my Braun Multipractic; this incredible tool is a hand-held blender, especially useful when the volume of a dish would require blending in several batches.
5 Process until quite smooth — you will still see some of the seeds from the eggplant, but that is fine.
6 Serve warm or (more commonly) at room temperature.

Makes 4 servings

Hummus

This is the wonderful, high-protein partner of baba ghanoush. To be truly authentic, place a little olive oil around the edges of the bowl before serving.

1 Sauté onion and garlic in oil until soft. Remove from heat.
2 Using a blender or food processor, puree chickpeas with remaining ingredients (except paprika).
3 Place in a serving bowl, and swirl decoratively with the back of a spoon.
4 Sprinkle with a little paprika and chill.
5 Serve chilled or at room temperature.

Makes 4 servings

Variation: add 2 tablespoons peanut or almond butter for a nutty hummus.

1 onion, peeled and minced
2 garlic cloves, minced
1 tablespoon olive oil
1 (16-ounce) can chickpeas,
    drained and rinsed
½ cup freshly squeezed lemon
    juice
¼ cup tahini
1–2 large green olives
Salt, pepper, and paprika
    (to taste)

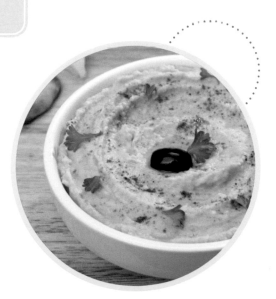

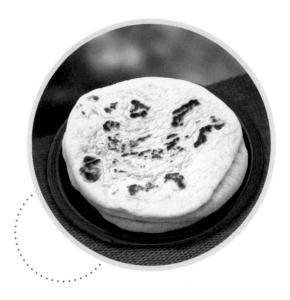

Indian Flatbread (Chapatis)

If your family ever eats curries or other Indian foods, this flatbread will complement the meal perfectly. Devised by the mother of an Indian celiac, it is very close to the real thing. Even if your family does not like Indian food, the bread makes a nice change of pace, is GF and yeast-free, and is easy to make on the stove top. You may need to find an Indo-Pak grocery store to get some of these ingredients — such stores have many unusual products you may want to try, and they nearly always carry Jowar flour. If you cannot find cilantro, you might want to grow it in your garden or in a window box. Cilantro makes a wonderful addition to Mexican foods as well.

2 cups rice flour

½ cup water, boiling

3 tablespoons fresh cilantro, chopped (many groceries carry this herb)

1 tablespoon green chilies, minced (canned chilies are very mild)

1 teaspoon curry leaves, chopped (these are not spicy)

½ teaspoon salt

2 tablespoons CF margarine, softened

1–2 tablespoons CF ghee (clarified butter, found in Indo-Pak stores) or oil

1 Mix flour with water, cilantro, chilies, and curry leaves. Add salt and margarine. Knead into a firm dough.

2 Divide dough into 8–10 balls and cover them with a damp tea towel or plastic wrap.

3 Heat a skillet to medium high and sprinkle some rice flour on a clean work surface.

4 Working with one ball at a time, flatten into a thin circle. To be perfectly authentic, use your hands, but if this is hard for you, a small rolling pin will do. Keep other dough balls covered while working.

5 Cook one flatbread at a time in a heavy skillet. When one side is dry, flip it over to cook the other side.

6 When slightly golden, drizzle with a few drops melted ghee.

7 Flip flatbread again so that the bottom also gets some fat.

Makes 4 servings

Pad Thai

This delicious noodle dish is a staple of Thai restaurants. If your family likes peanut butter, and noodles, you will probably have a hit on your hands. Although peanuts are traditional, you can use another nut and nut butter. If nuts are not tolerated, you could replace the nut butter with tahini.

1 Spoon peanut butter into a small dish and set aside.

2 Bring water to a boil in a pot. Add noodles and cook approximately 5 minutes or until noodles are soft.

3 Use boiling water, 1 tablespoon at a time, to thin the peanut butter until it can be poured.

4 Drain noodles and set aside.

5 Heat oil in a wok or large skillet over medium heat. Add garlic, scallions, and ginger, and stir-fry for approximately 2 minutes.

6 Add bok choy and stir-fry approximately 4 minutes. The vegetables should be tender, but still crispy.

7 Add the noodles, thinned peanut butter, and pepper to wok. Stir-fry until heated through.

8 Garnish with peanuts if desired. Serve immediately.

Makes 4 servings

¼ cup peanut butter

3 cups water

1 (7-ounce) package thin rice noodles (also called rice sticks)

2 tablespoons vegetable oil

1 garlic clove, minced

2 scallions, finely chopped

1 teaspoon fresh ginger, minced

2 cups shredded bok choy (or Chinese cabbage)

2 teaspoons GF tamari sauce

⅛ teaspoon pepper

Roasted peanuts, chopped (optional)

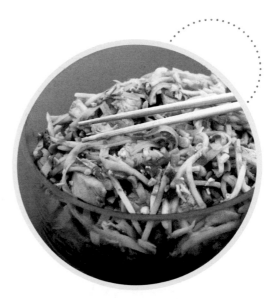

Picadillo

1 pound ground meat
   (preferably ground sirloin)
1 onion, minced
2 tomatoes, chopped
   (drained, canned tomatoes
   can be used)
1 garlic clove, minced
½ cup golden raisins
2 tablespoons apple cider
   vinegar
1 teaspoon sugar
1 teaspoon salt
1 teaspoon cinnamon
½ teaspoon cumin
½ teaspoon ground cloves
Pepper (to taste)
½ cup slivered almonds

I have no idea how authentic this recipe is. However, I was watching a new cooking show recently, and a Puerto Rican woman made it, so I guess it is "legit." I do know that almost everyone who tries it loves it. I have served it for family dinners and for company; it is always a big hit.

1 Brown meat in a pan and drain well.
2 Add onion and continue cooking until soft.
3 Add remaining ingredients (except almonds).
4 Stir mixture well and simmer over low heat for 20–30 minutes. Be careful not to burn it, and if necessary, add a few tablespoons water.
5 Spoon into a serving dish and top with almonds.
6 Serve with rice or corn bread.

Makes 4 servings

Hint: Decrease the amount of each spice if you want a milder dish.

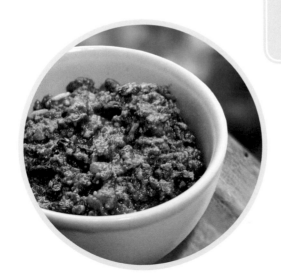

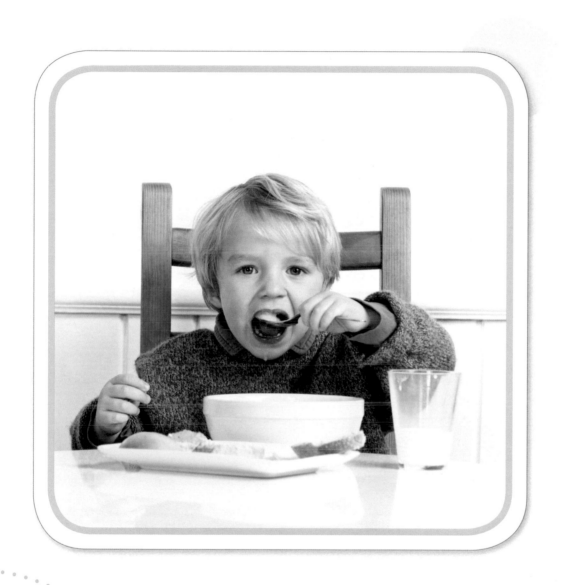

CHAPTER 12

Sweet Treats

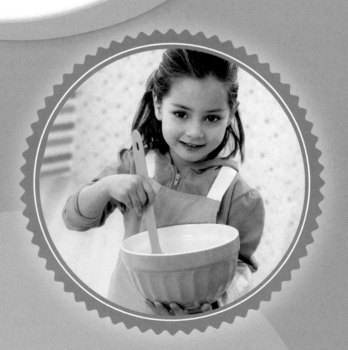

Sugar is not inherently evil, but most of us eat too much of it. In fact, it is currently estimated that the average American eats 150 pounds of sugar every year! Since there are many valid reasons for avoiding excess sugar, this is a real problem. Why do we have to avoid something we like so much? Well, sweets have three major strikes against them.

First, they are empty calories. If a child eats very little to begin with, or is extremely fussy, it is difficult to get the required nutrients on a daily basis. If the child has used up some of his small capacity on empty calories, it is nearly impossible.

Second, many children with autism have a demonstrable overgrowth of yeast. Sugar feeds yeast, so it must be strictly limited when trying to overcome this problem. Fortunately, in most cases a combination of diet, antifungal medication, and probiotic supplements eventually defeats the yeast problem. For some the problem can be persistent, however, and they really must avoid both refined and natural sugars for a time.

Finally, we all know our dentists hate sugar for the simple reason that it promotes tooth decay. The idea of trying to fill the teeth of children with autism is enough to scare the sugar out of most homes!

All that said, however, sweets taste good and children love them. I do believe that there is a place for sweets in the diet, albeit a small one. (Dieticians generally suggest that fewer than 10% of our daily calories come from refined sugars.)

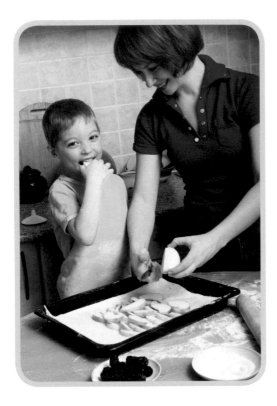

For really picky children, cookies and desserts present us with an opportunity for "sneaking in" nutrients that may otherwise be lacking in their diet. Growing children need between 800 and 1200 milligrams of calcium per day, for example, and for children who do not eat or drink dairy, it is sometimes hard to get the required amount. Powdered calcium is easily added to any of the recipes in this chapter, and I recommend you do so. A teaspoon of Kirkman Lab's powdered calcium contains

1,332 milligrams of this important mineral, and most recipes can take the addition of several teaspoons without a discernible change in texture. The powder is slightly sweet, however, so you may want to reduce your sweetener when using more than 1–2 teaspoons.

All children need the essential fatty acids (EFA), but few get them. Although flaxseed oil cannot be heated, ground flaxseed adds EFAs, as well as bulk and a delicious nutty flavor.. If you are searching for even more ways to get added protein into the diet, most cookies can take an extra egg or two. Extra egg helps add moisture and holds together cookies. Raisins and other dried fruits add both sweetness and nutrients (e.g., iron in raisins, calcium in figs).

For children who are fighting a yeast problem, intake of sugars must be drastically lowered. In fact, without substantial modification, most of the recipes in this chapter will be inappropriate for those on an anti-yeast regimen. However, there are sweetening ingredients that do not promote the growth of yeast, which may be used in moderation. These include the following:

- 100% pure food-grade vegetable glycerin
- Stevia
- Xylitol
- Lakanto

Vegetable glycerin is a thick, sweet, viscous liquid that is derived from coconut, and well tolerated by most people. It does not feed yeast, and can be used to sweeten many foods. It is easiest to substitute with glycerin when the original recipe calls for a liquid sweetener such as honey, molasses, or maple syrup. It is quite a bit sweeter than sugar, and you may have to experiment to get the amount right. If you do choose to use this liquid sweetener in a recipe that calls for regular sugar, you may need to decrease the liquid ingredients, and add something to make up for the bulk of the missing sugar. Always make sure that you buy "food-grade" vegetable glycerin; less pure forms are used in cosmetic products.

Stevia is an herb (*Stevia rebaudiana*) in the Chrysanthemum family. It grows wild as a small shrub in parts of Central and South America. The glycosides in its leaves, including up to 10% stevioside, account for its incredible sweetness. There are hundreds of species of stevia plants, but only the leaves of *S. rebaudiana* are used as a sweetener.

Stevia comes in several forms. The white powdered extract and the liquid extract are likely to be most useful to you when preparing foods. The green leaves are available in powdered form, but they tend to discolor

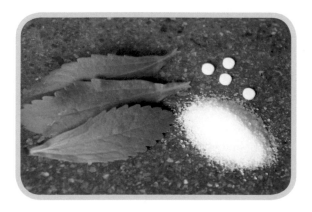

food. All stevia can have a bitter aftertaste; if too much is used, it will have a hint of licorice flavor. Many people who limit sugar have used stevia enthusiastically — others find it unpleasant tasting. I suggest you purchase a small amount at your local health food store and experiment. There are many recipes available at Stevia.com.

Bodyecology.com sells a liquid concentrate that has little of the "funny" stevia taste. A bottle costs about $20, but it will go a long way because it is so concentrated. Stevia is best used in drinks and other liquids — it really is not appropriate for baking.

Xylitol was discovered by a German chemist in 1891, and has been used as a sweetener in this country for nearly 40 years. Refined to a white crystalline powder, xylitol is odorless, with a pleasant, sweet taste. It has gained increasing acceptance as an alternative sweetener due to its role in reducing the development of dental cavities, and is often used to sweeten chewing gum.

Produced commercially from birch and other hardwood trees, xylitol has the same sweetness and bulk as sugar with one-third fewer calories and no unpleasant aftertaste. This means that it can be used, cup for cup, as you would use sugar. It dissolves quickly, and may produce an odd yet pleasant cooling sensation in the mouth.

Xylitol is sold in several forms and under many names. One brand called "The Ultimate Sweetener" in available in both granular and powdered form. Many natural food stores

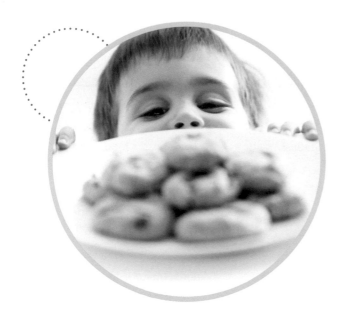

for cup like sugar, tastes terrific, and does not feed yeast. It has no additives and does not affect blood sugar or insulin release. On the downside — it is really expensive. As of this writing, Lakanto retails for almost $20 per pound.

Of course, if you really only bake for very special occasions, it might be worth it to have a really good result for your family members who are on a sugar-limited diet. Only you can decide if you want to splurge in this way, but it is a great product.

Lakanto is made from a fermented sugar alcohol called erythritol, and a sweet extract of a Chinese fruit called luo han guo. Erythritol is found naturally in grapes, pears, mushrooms, and other foods. Unlike other sugar alcohols (e.g., sorbitol, malitol), the erythritol in Lakanto does not cause diarrhea, gas, or bloating — probably because it has been fermented. Other sugar alcohols are made from hydrogenation. The erythritol in Lakanto is fermented from non-GMO corn, so it is possible (though unlikely) that people sensitive to corn might react to it.

Some companies are now selling erythritol alone as a sweetener, but without the luo han guo, it does not really taste like sugar.

Experiment with substituting sugar alternatives in the recipes in this chapter and in your family's favorites. You may also want to use a combination of a little sugar and one of the substitutes. This will appreciably lessen the amount of sugar being consumed while reducing any unusual flavor or aftertaste.

carry it, as do online stores. Xylitol should be well tolerated by anyone not allergic to birch bark. It does not feed yeast, and is appropriate for most yeast-free diets.

In general, if you are avoiding sugar in your family's diet, I would say that xylitol makes an excellent overall substitute. Because you can use it as a cup-for-cup substitute, adding extra bulk to a recipe is not necessary. On the downside, it is expensive, at approximately $9 per pound. However, if your child must be on a sugar-free diet, it is probably worth the expense to be able to provide an occasional cookie!

Lakanto is the new kid on the sugar-substitute block. Available from Bodyecology.com, Lakanto has many things going for it and makes an excellent substitute for sugar when you are baking occasional treats. What makes it so great? It has zero calories, measures cup

A Few Words about Artificial Sweeteners

I do not advocate or support the use of artificial sweeteners such as sucralose (Splenda) or aspartame (NutraSweet and Equal). Studies have shown that these artificial ingredients can have neurological and other ill effects. According to Dr. Joseph Mercola (www. mercola.com), "... sucralose is a chlorocarbon. The chlorocarbons have long been known for causing organ, genetic, and reproductive damage. It should be no surprise, therefore, that the testing of sucralose reveals that it can cause up to 40% shrinkage of the thymus: a gland that is the very foundation of our immune system."

Aspartame is even worse. It is made up of three chemicals: phenylalanine, aspartic acid, and methanol (wood alcohol). The first two chemicals are amino acids that are harmless when ingested as food. However, in aspartame they are combined with an ester bond. When the body breaks down this bond, there can be neurotoxic effects from the free amino acids. Headaches, mental confusion, and even seizures have been reported. The high concentration of these chemicals in the form of aspartame floods your central nervous system and can cause excessive firing of brain neurons, a condition known as *excitotoxicity*.

The elements of aspartame itself are not necessarily harmful, but they become toxic when metabolized. If you are interested in a full explanation, I suggest you visit Dr.

Mercola's website and do a search on aspartame. For now, suffice it to say that your family can and should live without it!

One last note about ingredients — I use a lot of peanut butter! It is a nutrient-dense food that most children love, and it adds moisture and fat to a recipe. I realize, however, that many children cannot tolerate peanuts. Any nut butter will work in recipes that specify peanut butter. Remember that peanuts are legumes — a peanut intolerance does not

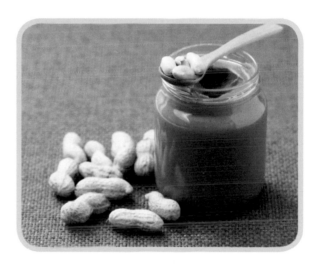

mean that tree nuts are unacceptable (though for allergic children, they might not be appropriate). Do not forget to try the more unusual nut butters such as pistachio and macadamia. If you fear cross-contamination, it is simple to make your own nut butter if you have a high-powered blender or a good food processor. If your child cannot tolerate any nut, tahini often makes a good substitute. Made from sesame seeds, tahini adds a similar taste and texture, and has the added benefit of being another source of calcium.

You may want to reread the sections on flours and baking techniques in chapter 5. I recommend you experiment with flours, nuts, dried fruits, chips, and other add-ins. Use what your family likes. Be creative and experiment.

Baking cookies is a wonderful way to spend time with your child. Even the most distractible child will get interested in this kind of activity—and many a speech or math lesson has been taught while mixing, stirring, measuring, and pouring. Little fingers can be taught to crack eggs, and little hands are good at stirring. So pull up a stool, tie on the aprons, let the GF flour fly, and make cookies!

Note: I usually use the standard Hagman blend of rice flour, potato starch flour, and tapioca starch flour when a recipe calls for GF flour. There are many other formulas and many GF flour blends available commercially. Use the blend that you prefer. Many recipes will work with almond or other nut flours if grains are removed from the diet.

Cakes

For most of our children, cakes are and should be for special occasions only. Birthdays and major holidays are the only times you will want to consult this section. That said, it really is a nice thing to do for these special occasions, and by making and serving cakes infrequently you ensure that they are special.

When I wrote *Special Diets for Special Kids*, there were very few options other than baking from scratch. No grocery store carried appropriate cakes, and there were very few mixes available. For that reason, the first two editions included many recipes for cakes. Now, things have really changed. Even the venerable Betty Crocker has a line of GF mixes! (Check the ingredient lists, but many do not contain too many additives and should be fine for occasional use.) I generally bake from scratch, and I have included a few cake recipes here. There are times, however, when it is extremely handy to have a good mix on the shelf. I always have one or two on hand. When something comes up and I need to provide a cake or cupcakes, I can do it quickly. ★

Pineapple Velvet Cake

2½ cups GF flour mix

1 tablespoon GF baking
    powder

2 teaspoons xanthan gum

1 teaspoon baking soda

½ teaspoon salt

4 eggs

1 cup vegetable oil

1⅔ cups sugar

2 teaspoons fresh lemon juice

1 teaspoon pure vanilla extract

1 cup unsweetened pineapple
    juice

Lynne Davis created this recipe many years ago. I almost left it out, but it has become such a classic of the GFCF repertoire that I figured I would include it for anyone who has not seen it in my book or online. (Do a Google search and you will find it has been reproduced many times and in many places!) Pineapple juice is tolerated by most people, and adds a lovely flavor without being overpowering. This makes a wonderful cake or cupcakes.

Lynne uses a simple pineapple glaze, which is delicious, but since the cake is very moist (and we want to reduce sugar) it does not need frosting. If desired, dust the top of the finished cake with 1 tablespoon confectioner's sugar, sifted through a tea strainer or other fine mesh.

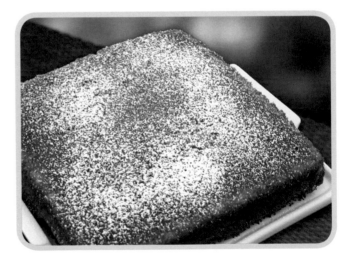

1 Preheat the oven to 350°F.

2 Combine dry ingredients, and set aside.

3 With an electric mixer, blend eggs, oil, sugar, lemon juice, and vanilla. Beat well so oil is completely emulsified, and mixture is light and lemony looking.

4 Turn beater to low, and add dry mixture and pineapple juice, alternating.

5 Pour batter into greased and floured tins: 1 (9"x13") pan, 2 (9" round) cake pans, or cupcake tins.

6 Bake for 25–30 minutes for cakes, or 15–20 minutes for cupcakes.

Servings will vary.

Variation: As stated above, this is a versatile recipe. It has a lovely texture, and can be modified for nearly any flavor you want. Simply replace juice in recipe with another flavor juice, or with liquid milk substitute (to start with a more neutral base). For example, to make a maple cake, you might replace some of sugar with pure, granulated maple sugar (available at gourmet shops and through mail order). Then use natural maple flavoring in place of vanilla, and flavor frosting to suit the cake.

✳ Zebra Cake

1 or 2-layer yellow cake batter, from scratch or GFCF mix
2 tablespoons unsweetened cocoa for each layer
Confectioner's sugar (optional)

The zebra cake is a fun thing to make, and the "stripes" add so much interest that extra adornment (like frosting) is completely unnecessary. I dust this cake with a little confectioner's sugar or some plain cocoa. The minute you slice into it, all eyes are on the inside of the cake! This really is not a recipe, but rather a technique. I usually make this as a 9″ one-layer cake.

1 Divide cake batter into 2 bowls. Set one bowl aside, and in the other sift in cocoa. Use a whisk to mix well — you do not want lumps.

2 Prepare your pan(s) with baking spray or oil. Spoon batter into pan, alternating chocolate and plain. Start with plain batter, and spoon about 2 tablespoons (I use a large serving spoon or a ¼ cup measure) into center of pan. Add same amount of chocolate batter directly on top of the first spoonful. Continue in this manner, always placing batter in center of previous spoonful.

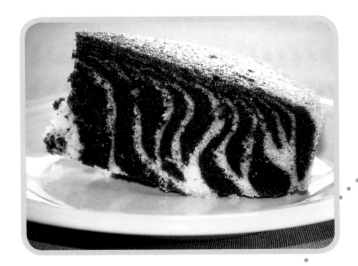

3 At first, you will have batter in the middle of pan, but as you continue, the weight of batter will push it out to sides of pan. The two colors will form concentric circles (see picture). Do not worry if they are not perfect!

4 Bake cake according to your recipe or mix directions.

5 If cake has formed a pronounced peak, you may want to use a breadknife to slice it off before you turn cake onto a serving plate.

6 Let cake cool completely. Dust with confectioner's sugar or cocoa (or a mixture of both).

7 Slice cake when cool, and prepare to wow your guests!

Servings will vary.

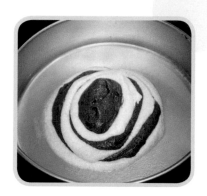

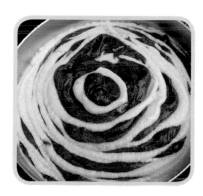

Variation: You can add food coloring instead of cocoa to make colored stripes. Pink stripes might thrill little girls at a birthday party. Be sure to use natural colors (visit www.naturesflavors.com, or http://organic. lovetoknow.com/Natural_Food_Coloring). Using orange for the "plain" color, and cocoa for the dark, will turn this into a tiger cake!

✴ Flourless Chocolate Cake

8 ounces good quality
   bittersweet chocolate
1 cup CF margarine
1½ cups sugar
1⅛ cups cocoa powder,
   divided
6 eggs

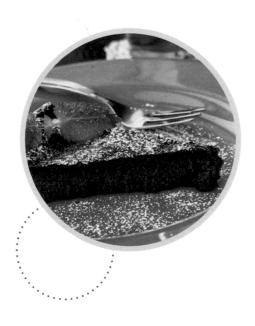

This is my "go-to" cake these days. It is easy to put together, and since it is not supposed to have flour, there are few modifications needed for a really rich, wonderful dessert. It is very dense, and should be sliced into small pieces. There is no leavening in this cake, and it will not rise very much (and if it does rise a little, it will fall!). Do not worry about its appearance — sift a little cocoa or confectioner's sugar on top and sprinkle some berries around the sides. No one will mind the way it looks. I always serve this with fresh raspberries.

1 Preheat oven to 375°F.

2 Grease a 9″ springform pan, and line bottom with a circle of wax paper or parchment, cut to fit. Grease again.

3 Melt chocolate and margarine over low heat, and cool slightly.

4 Sift sugar and 1 cup cocoa together in a bowl. Whisk eggs lightly in another bowl.

5 Add eggs to dry ingredients, and whisk together until well mixed.

6 Add margarine and chocolate mixture to egg mixture. Be sure that chocolate has cooled a bit so that you do not scramble eggs.

7 Mix well and scrape batter into prepared pan.

8 Bake cake in middle of oven for about 25 minutes, or until a thin crust has formed on top.

9 Cool cake in its pan for 5 minutes before inverting on a plate.

10 Carefully remove sides of pan, and dust top of cake with a sifting of remaining cocoa.

Makes 1 (9″) cake

Farfel "Cake"

This is not a cake, nor does it contain farfel (matzo crumbs). It is a recipe given to me years ago by a grad school friend, Michele Blum. I am often asked for this recipe — and it is so easy I am almost embarrassed to share it! This pat-in crust can be used for any fruit pie. **Hint:** Be sure to use a large enough pan (9"–10") so that your crust will be thin.

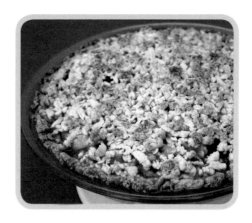

1 Cream margarine, sugar, and oil. Add remaining ingredients (except pie filling), and mix well.

2 Divide dough (it will be soft) in half. Wrap one-half in plastic, and place in refrigerator until firm. Pat other half into bottom and sides of a 10" pie or quiche pan to make crust.

3 Fill crust with pie filling.

4 Grate second half of dough on top of filling, forming a streusel topping.

5 Bake for 1 hour at 350°F, or until golden brown.

Servings will vary.

½ cup CF margarine

½ cup sugar

1 tablespoon vegetable oil

2 eggs, beaten

2 cups GF flour

2 teaspoons pure vanilla extract

2 teaspoons xanthan gum

2 teaspoons GF baking powder

1 (15.5-ounce) can fruit pie filling (or 5 cups chopped fruit mixed with ¼ cup sugar and 2 tsp cinnamon)

Variation: For a simple, mock linzer torte, exchange ¼ cup GF flour for ¼ cup almond or pecan meal, and use raspberry jam to fill. You will get raves, I promise!

✸ Buckwheat Cake

I cup buckwheat flour

I cup, minus 3 tablespoons
   GF flour blend

½ teaspoon cinnamon

I teaspoon sea salt, divided
   (I always use French Fleur
   De Sel, but any coarse,
   grained sea salt will work)

I cup Earth Balance
   shortening, softened
   (or other dairy-free oleo)

I cup sugar

I whole egg

5 egg yolks, divided

I teaspoon pure vanilla extract

I tablespoon prepared coffee

I teaspoon milk substitute

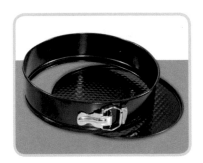

A few years ago, we visited northern France. My husband has relatives in Brittany, and we wanted to visit some of the World War II sites in Normandy. We were stunned by the wonderful food, and how different it was from (also wonderful) Parisian food. Buckwheat and butter features very prominently in much of the cuisine in this region, and we had a delicious buckwheat cake that I really wanted to duplicate. I was not sure where to start, but then one of my favorite authors and food bloggers, David Liebovitz, published a similar cake in his marvelous book, *The Sweet Life in Paris*. His cake is full of sweet butter and wheat flour, but it inspired this version. It is delicious — and looks beautiful too.

1 Preheat oven to 350°F.

2 Use cooking spray to generously coat bottom and sides of a 9" springform pan. (You will want to use pan with a removable bottom.)

3 Sift flours together with cinnamon and ½ teaspoon salt.

4 Using an electric mixer, beat shortening until fluffy, then add sugar and continue beating until light.

5 In another bowl, beat 4 egg yolks and I whole egg with vanilla and coffee.

6 Gradually add egg mixture to batter while continuing to beat. Beat until it is very fluffy.

7 Mix dry ingredients into batter. Try not to overmix, but be sure it is well incorporated.

8 Use a rubber spatula to scrape batter into pan. Smooth top with a knife or an offset (angled) spatula.

9 Mix I egg yolk and milk substitute together in a small bowl to create glaze.

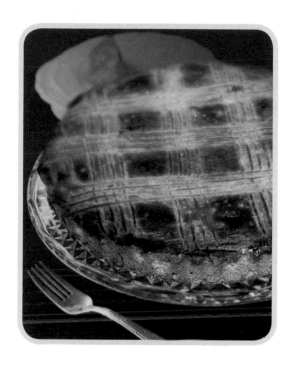

10 Brush glaze over top of cake. (You will use most of it.)

11 Use a fork to make a crisscross pattern across top of cake, then sprinkle with about ⅓ teaspoon sea salt.

12 Bake cake for 45 minutes. Do not overbake, or cake will dry out.

Makes 8–10 servings

One-Bowl Chocolate Cake

1½ cups GF flour mix

1 cup sugar

3 tablespoons unsweetened cocoa

2 teaspoons xanthan gum

1 teaspoon GF baking soda

½ teaspoon salt

5 tablespoons vegetable oil

1 teaspoon pure vanilla extract

1 teaspoon vinegar

1 cup cold water

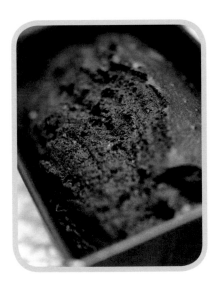

This type of cake was made popular by Peg Bracken in the 1988 book, *The Compleat I Hate to Cook Book*. Versions of this "wacky" or "cockeyed" cake have been around for years, and this is a GF version. It is not the world's best cake, but it is very moist and whips up with very little fuss or cleanup. It is also egg-free. Baking without eggs is tricky, and for those who must avoid eggs, finding a cake recipe is not easy. In some versions of the cake recipe, you mix it right in the baking pan, making separate wells for each liquid ingredient. I find that one well is sufficient, and the cake bakes more evenly if mixed in a bowl and then poured into the prepared pan. **Note:** I suggest using the traditional Hagman GF flour mix, rather than a mixture that contains bean flours.

1 Preheat oven to 350°F.

2 In a large mixing bowl, sift flour, sugar, cocoa, xanthan gum, baking soda, and salt.

3 Make a well in flour mixture, and put in oil, vanilla, and vinegar. Pour cold water over mixture, and stir until moistened.

4 Pour batter into a greased 8" square pan.

5 Bake for 25–30 minutes, or until cake springs back when touched lightly.

Makes 1 (8") cake

Fruit Cobbler

My sister gave me this recipe years ago, and I found it works just as well with the GF flour mixture. This dessert is perfect for fruit just starting to darken but too good to throw away. If possible, serve it warm from the oven. Adjust the sweetening to the fruit — only very tart fruit should need the full ½ cup sugar mixed in. A mixture of fruit works especially well.

5 cups fruit (e.g., berries, sliced pears, apples, plums, peaches)

1 cup sugar (or equivalent amount of preferred sweetener), divided

½ cup, plus 2 tablespoons GF flour, divided

1 tablespoon lemon juice

1 teaspoon pure vanilla extract

½ teaspoon cinnamon

1 egg, beaten

2 tablespoons CF margarine, melted

½ teaspoon GF baking powder

1 Place a sheet of aluminum foil on bottom of oven — this is very messy!

2 Preheat oven to 375°F.

3 Mix fruit with ½ cup sugar, 2 tablespoons flour, lemon juice, vanilla, and cinnamon. Toss until fruit is evenly coated.

4 Place mixture in a 2-quart casserole or baking dish. Dot with margarine, if desired.

5 Mix egg, ½ cup flour, ½ cup sugar, margarine, and baking powder to make topping.

6 Spoon topping onto fruit, covering as much of fruit mixture as possible (it does not have to be perfectly covered).

7 Bake until cobbler topping is golden, approximately 45–50 minutes.

Makes 6-8 servings

Variations: If you like a topping with a crumbly texture, add ¼–½ cup ground pecans or almonds.

During winter, use apple or pears together with fresh or frozen cranberries. Add a few golden raisins, and you have a wonderful dessert.

Puddings

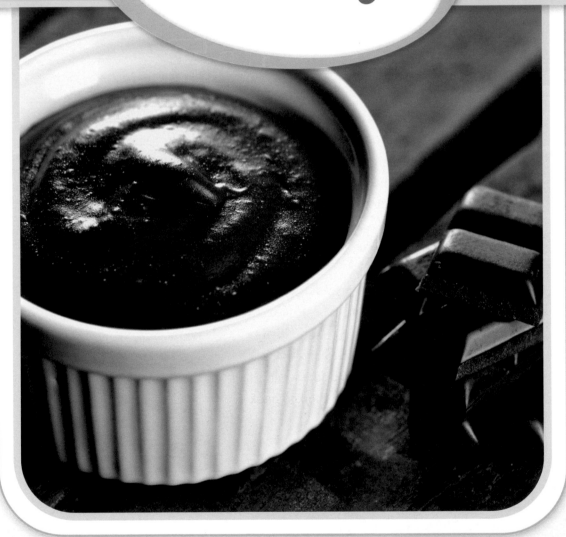

Chocolate Pudding (or Pie Filling), recipe on page 304

✳ Tapioca Pudding

There is no middle ground with tapioca pudding — it is a love or hate thing. It has kind of a weird, bumpy texture that is either irritating or enjoyable in the mouth. I have always loved it, and it is a quick, easy pudding to make from scratch. There are lots of ways to vary it — add dried fruit like raisins, or any fresh fruit you like. A little cocoa makes chocolate tapioca pudding. This version uses coconut — it is great as written, but try adding bananas, mango, or another tropical fruit for a real treat.

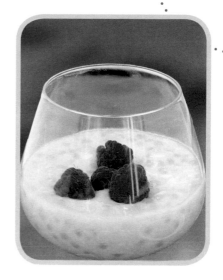

1 Bring water to boil and add tapioca. Whisk pearls to keep them from clumping.

2 Lower heat and cook tapioca for 15 minutes. As pearls give up their starch, they become clearer and water becomes thick and viscous. Stir occasionally to keep pearls from sticking.

3 In a separate bowl, combine coconut milk, agave, vanilla, and salt.

4 When tapioca is done, whisk liquid mixture into saucepan and simmer for 5 minutes.

5 Add shredded coconut if desired, and cook for 3 more minutes.

6 Refrigerate and serve cold. Stir well before serving. If tapioca has gotten solid at bottom, use a fork to break it up, then stir until smooth.

4 cups water
6 tablespoons small pearl
    tapioca
1½ cups coconut milk
    (or almond milk)
4 tablespoons agave nectar
    (or honey)
1 teaspoon pure vanilla extract
¼ teaspoon salt
⅔ cup unsweetened, shredded
    coconut (optional)

Makes 4 servings

Variation: Top with a dollop of sweetened cashew cream.

✦new✦ Chocolate Pudding (or Pie Filling)

¼ cup sugar

2 tablespoons tapioca starch flour

1 teaspoon espresso powder (optional)

2 cups coconut milk (or almond milk)

1 cup semisweet GFCF chocolate chips

1½ tablespoons pure vanilla extract

1 tablespoon CF margarine (I like Earth Balance)

Everyone loves chocolate pudding! This is a really good recipe that is not too sweet. It is easy to make and could be used in a pie if you are so inclined. Coffee deepens the flavor of chocolate, though you will not taste it. You can leave it out if you prefer.

1 Whisk sugar, tapioca starch flour, and espresso powder in a heavy saucepan.

2 Turn heat to medium, and gradually whisk in coconut milk. Continue whisking until mixture boils and starts to thicken, about 5 minutes.

3 Remove saucepan from heat, and stir in chocolate chips, margarine, and vanilla until smooth.

4 Divide mixture between 6 small cups. Cover each with plastic wrap, pressed lightly on the surface to prevent a skin from forming.

5 Chill for about 2 hours.

Makes 6 servings

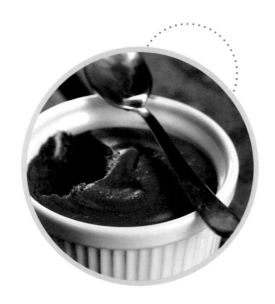

Pies

Many children strongly prefer cakes and cupcakes to pie, but there are times (such as Thanksgiving or Christmas) when you really want to make a pie. My strategy is always to make a pie that everyone can eat, rather than "special" versus "regular" crusts. If the crust and filling are good enough, no one will care if it contains gluten or not.

The problem is, making good GF piecrust is a bit of a challenge. Piecrust just seems to cry out for gluten, and most people really do not want to bother with making it.

In past editions, I included piecrust recipes because there were no other options. Now, however, there are excellent mixes available from Glutino, Allergy Free Grocer, and other companies. Whole Foods even makes an excellent frozen GF pie crust (though as of this writing it is not dairy-free).

Another option is to make a refrigerator pie using a cracker- or cookie-crumb crust. Though I do not make pies often, this is how I most commonly do it. And if you really want to cut back on starches, some pies (e.g., pumpkin) can be baked without any crust at all by pouring the filling into ramekins and baking. If you like the idea of making a refrigerator pie instead of a rolled piecrust, here are some alternatives. **Note:** There is also a Ginger Snap Crust recipe in Chapter 9. ★

"Graham" Cracker Crust

1 (7.5-ounce) package Healthy
    Valley Rice Bran crackers,
    blended or processed to
    crumbs
¼ cup sugar
¼ cup CF margarine, softened
½ teaspoon cinnamon
    (optional)

Health Valley makes a wonderful ersatz graham cracker called Rice Bran Crackers. They are available at health food stores and some groceries.

1 Preheat oven to 350°F.
2 Combine all ingredients in a large mixing bowl. Mix until well blended.
3 Place crumbs in a 9" pie pan, and press into bottom and up sides of pan.
4 Bake crust for 6–8 minutes, until slightly toasted.
5 Cool slightly before spooning in cooked pie filling.

Makes 1 pie crust

Variations: Flaked coconut (sulfite-free) makes a good addition to this crust. Use ¼ cup pecan or almond meal to enhance a graham crust.

For banana pie, line bottom of crust with sliced bananas prior to filling with vanilla custard or pudding. Toss additional slices of banana with lemon juice to prevent browning, and place a border of sliced banana around circumference of pie.

✳ Cookie-Crumb Crust

The beauty of a cookie-crumb crust (besides the part about not rolling it out!) is that you can use any kind of cookie you want. For some fillings, you might want to use chocolate wafer cookies (see recipe on page 310). For others you might want to use a ginger snap, vanilla cookie, or even a macaroon. If your child is on a grain-free diet, you can use the SCD cookie from page 313. The process is always the same. You can crumb your cookies in a food processor or blender, or you can go low tech — put cookies in a strong bag and use a rolling pin to break into crumbs.

1 Preheat oven to 375°F.
2 Mix cookie crumbs, sugar, and margarine in a bowl; it should have consistency of wet sand.
3 Press crumb mixture up against sides and bottom of a 9" pie pan. (You can use your hands, but a straight-sided shot glass can be helpful. I have a tiny little rolling pin that I use for this task.)
4 Bake for 10–15 minutes, or until it just starts to brown.
5 Cool completely before spooning in filling.

Makes 1 pie crust

1½ cups cookie crumbs
¼ cup sugar
(use honey for SCD)
¼ cup margarine, melted
(or shortening or ghee)

Cookies

A word about servings. Most cookbooks tell you how many cookies the recipe will make. I have included an approximate number of cookies to expect from each recipe. It depends on how large you make cookies. I prefer them big, so I routinely get a dozen fewer than the recipe amount. If you like small cookies, you will get more. In general, a recipe that calls for 2 cups flour will yield about 24 big cookies, or 36 small cookies. If a recipe calls for 3 or more cups flour — add another 12 cookies to the yield. ⋆

Panda Puff
Chocolate Crisps

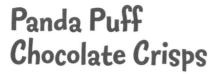

First, Envirokiz came up with Gorilla Munch cereal, then Panda Puffs, and now they have added Leapin' Lemurs! All these cereals are delicious and make excellent cookies. Use the variety of your choice for this popular recipe. I first made them with Gorilla Munch, but since Panda Puffs are already peanut butter flavored, it was a natural. All three cereals are corn-based and contain soy, so they may not be appropriate for your kids.

1 Preheat oven to 325°F.

2 Stir peanut butter, sugars, margarine, baking soda, baking powder, and egg in a large bowl until well mixed. Fold in cereal and chocolate chips.

3 Shape dough by rounded tablespoonfuls into balls; place about 2" apart on an ungreased baking sheet (do not crowd them as these cookies tend to spread).

4 Bake cookies for 10–12 minutes, or until golden brown.

5 Cool 5 minutes, then remove cookies from the baking sheet.

6 Cool completely. Store loosely covered.

Servings will vary.

½ cup peanut butter
⅓ cup granulated sugar
⅓ cup brown sugar, packed
⅓ cup CF margarine, softened
½ teaspoon GF baking soda
½ teaspoon GF baking powder
I egg, beaten
4 cups Envirokiz cereal
I cup GFCF semisweet
  chocolate chips

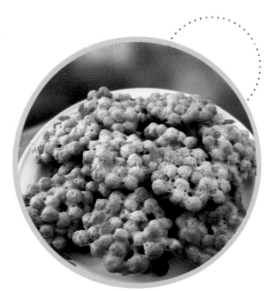

Chocolate Wafers

1 (18-ounce) GFCF chocolate
   cake mix
½ cup GF flour blend
3 tablespoons shortening,
   melted
1 egg, beaten
¼ cup water, divided

These plain wafer cookies are really good, and they can easily be turned into a Thin Mint-type cookie. Well worth the trouble!

1 Combine first four ingredients in a large bowl, adding water a little at a time until dough forms.
2 Gather dough into a ball, wrap tightly, and refrigerate for at least 2 hours.
3 Preheat oven to 350°F.
4 On a GF flour–covered surface, roll out dough, a portion at a time, to no thicker than ¹⁄₁₆". You want very thin cookies! Cut into very small cookies, 1½" diameter (if you do not have a cutter that small, use the lid from a spice jar).
5 Bake cookies on a lightly greased cookie sheet for approximately 10 minutes.

Makes 36 cookies

Making Thin Mints

1 Melt chocolate chips with shortening in a saucepan over low heat.

2 When chocolate is completely melted, add peppermint oil (not extract), and stir well.

3 Using a fork (or special dipping tool available in candy making supply stores), dip each cooled chocolate wafer into chocolate mixture.

4 Let excess chocolate drip off, and place cookies on wax paper.

5 When chocolate hardens enough to touch cookies, place them on wax paper-covered baking sheets.

6 Chill cookies until completely firm. Wrap well and store in refrigerator or freezer.

1 (12-ounce) bag GFCF
  chocolate chips
1 tablespoon shortening
2 drops peppermint oil*
Chocolate Wafers (see recipe
  on page 310)

 *Peppermint oil can be found in cake and candy making supply stores; it is very strong, so do not use more than 2 drops!

✸ Charlie's Macaroons

3 egg whites

Pinch salt

½ cup white sugar (to taste)

½ cup almonds, chopped and
toasted

½ cup GFCF chocolate chips
(optional)

1 (5-ounce) package
unsweetened, shredded
coconut

2 tablespoons brown rice flour

1 teaspoon pure vanilla extract

Sometimes when I speak to local groups, Charlie Fall comes with me. She does nutritional counseling with parents and has lots of good advice, and it is a good networking opportunity for everyone. Once she brought along these fantastic cookies, and I had to have the recipe. They are easy, delicious, and addictive. They are sweet, and should be an occasional treat only. The cookies freeze well — if there are any left!

1 Preheat oven to 325°F.

2 Beat egg whites and salt until loosely foamy and opaque. Add remaining ingredients.

3 Form balls from mixture by hand or use a cookie scoop. If texture is too loose, add a little more rice flour. If a few chocolate chips escape, push ball together with your hands.

4 Bake cookies on a non-stick baking sheet for 10–12 minutes.

5 Cool cookies on a rack and enjoy.

Servings will vary.

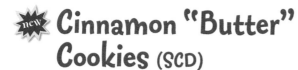 # Cinnamon "Butter" Cookies (SCD)

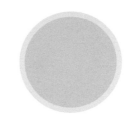

This is another recipe from Pam Ferro of the Gottschall Center in Massachusetts. It is appropriate for anyone following the SCD or other restricted carbohydrate diet, and very tasty too. This cookie is also delicious frozen and eaten straight from the freezer!

2 cups almond flour
½ cup ghee
⅓ cup honey
2 teaspoons cinnamon
½ teaspoon sea salt
¼ teaspoon GF baking soda

1 Preheat oven to 300°F.
2 Combine all ingredients in a mixing bowl.
3 Form dough into 1" diameter balls on a greased baking sheet.
4 Bake cookies for 10 minutes.

Makes 30 cookies

The Best GF Chocolate Chip Cookies

1½ cups white rice flour*

½ cup sweet rice flour*

¼ cup potato starch*

2 teaspoons xanthan gum

1 teaspoon GF baking soda

1 teaspoon salt

½ teaspoon GF baking powder

½ cup sugar

½ cup brown sugar, packed

1 cup CF margarine

2 eggs

1 teaspoon pure vanilla extract

1 (12-ounce) package GFCF
chocolate chips

1 cup walnuts, chopped
(optional)

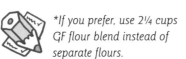

*If you prefer, use 2¼ cups
GF flour blend instead of
separate flours.

Have you ever met someone who did not love chocolate chip cookies? I certainly have not! There are lots of decent mixes and prepared cookies around, but nothing is quite as good as a homemade cookie. This is the same recipe I have published before, but with an important difference. This dough should be made at least 1 day ahead, and allowed to chill overnight. Some cookie experts say that chocolate cookie dough should be chilled for 2–3 days before baking. Even Mrs. Wakefield, sainted inventor of the cookie at the Toll House Inn, refrigerated her dough overnight. By letting the dough rest, you enable it to soak up the liquid ingredients. This gives you a firmer, drier dough, and leads to a cookie with a much better texture. The bottom line is that you can bake this cookie right away, but if you can hold off for 1–2 days, you will be rewarded with a more delicious cookie!

1 Combine dry ingredients in a small bowl. Set aside.

2 Cream sugars and margarine until well blended. Beat in eggs, one at a time. Add vanilla.

3 Gradually add flour mixture to liquid mixture, and mix well. Fold in chocolate chips and nuts.

4 Refrigerate dough overnight.

5 When ready to bake, preheat oven to 375°F.

6 Drop by rounded teaspoonfuls on an ungreased baking sheet.

7 Bake cookies for 10–12 minutes.

8 Cool on a wire rack.

Makes 36 cookies

Variation: To make chocolate-chocolate chip cookies, replace ¼ cup rice flour with ½ cup unsweetened cocoa.

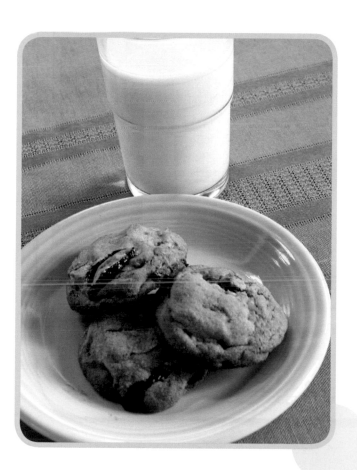

⭐ *new* Chewy Chocolate Cookies

3 cups powdered sugar

½ cup good quality, unsweetened cocoa

2 tablespoons GF flour

3 egg whites

2 cups pecans, chopped and toasted

These are delicious cookies — rich and chewy. The original recipe called for only 2 tablespoons flour, and they work just as well with GF flour. They are very sweet so make them for special occasions only.

1 Preheat oven to 350°F.

2 Line 2 baking sheets with parchment, non-stick foil, or silicone baking mats.

3 Combine sugar, cocoa, and flour in bowl of an electric mixer, and beat until well mixed.

4 Beat in egg whites, one at a time. Scrape bowl as necessary to fully combine, then beat on high speed for 1 minute. Fold pecans into mixture.

5 Drop mixture in heaping tablespoonfuls onto prepared sheets. Leave 2″ between cookies, as they will spread.

6 Bake cookies for 15 minutes in center of oven, turning front to back halfway through baking.

7 Cool completely, then carefully peel cookies off pan liner.

8 Store cookies in an airtight container or freeze.

Servings will vary.

World's Easiest Chocolate Cookies

Everyone has a recipe for these little brownie-like cookies. Usually they are rolled in powdered sugar before baking and called "Krinkles" or "Crackles." They do not need extra sugar, and taste the same without the messy extra step. I decided to see if I could make them really fast using a GF cookie mix. I did, and I have to admit to being a little miffed when my husband ate one and said it was the best chocolate cookie I had made in ages! With three ingredients, this hardly qualifies as a "recipe," but give it a go and try not to blush over the praise you will receive.

1 (18-ounce) package GFCF chocolate cake mix
¼ cup oil
2 eggs, beaten

1 Preheat oven to 350°F.
2 Combine cake mix, oil, and eggs until well mixed.
3 Shape dough into walnut-sized balls, and place on lightly greased (or parchment lined) baking sheet.
4 Bake cookies for 10 minutes, or until set.
5 Cool for 10 minutes before moving cookies to wire racks.

Makes 36 cookies

Pignoli Cookies

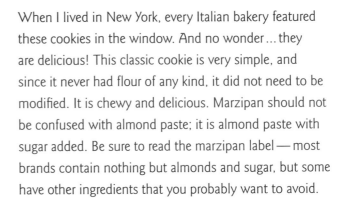

1¼ cups (9 ounces) marzipan
½ cup almond flour
¼ cup sugar
1 teaspoon almond extract
⅛ teaspoon salt
2–3 drops lemon oil
1 large egg white
1½ cups pine nuts (pignoli)

When I lived in New York, every Italian bakery featured these cookies in the window. And no wonder... they are delicious! This classic cookie is very simple, and since it never had flour of any kind, it did not need to be modified. It is chewy and delicious. Marzipan should not be confused with almond paste; it is almond paste with sugar added. Be sure to read the marzipan label — most brands contain nothing but almonds and sugar, but some have other ingredients that you probably want to avoid.

1 Preheat oven to 325°F.
2 Lightly grease (or line with parchment) 2 baking sheets.
3 Break marzipan into pieces into a medium bowl. Mix in flour, sugar, almond extract, salt, and lemon oil; the mixture will be crumbly. Add egg white, beating until mixture is smooth.
4 Place pine nuts in a shallow dish. Using a teaspoon cookie scoop, or your lightly oiled or wet hands, drop 1" balls of dough into pine nuts, rolling and pressing gently to coat them thoroughly. (You may also simply grab a handful of pine nuts, and roll dough between your palms, pressing in pine nuts as you go; the point is to cover dough with nuts.)
5 Place cookies on baking sheets, leaving about 1" between them.
6 Bake cookies for 22–24 minutes, or until lightly browned.
7 Cool cookies on sheets for 5 minutes, then transfer to a rack to cool completely.

Makes 26 cookies

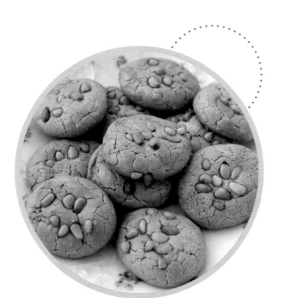

More Sweet Treats

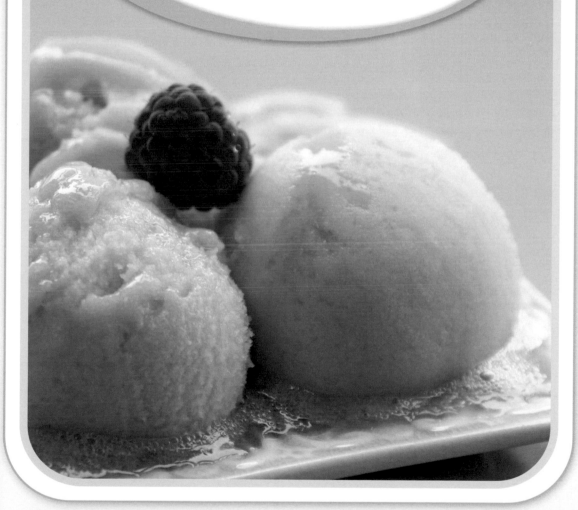

SCD Orange Sorbet, recipe on page 320

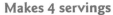 SCD Orange Sorbet

1 cup simple syrup
   (equal parts honey and
   water, simmered until honey
   is completely dissolved)
1 cup unsweetened orange
   juice
¼ cup water
1 teaspoon lemon juice

Sorbets are easy to find at the grocery store, but most commercially available sorbets contain corn syrup, and all contain sugar. If you are following the SCD, this version will work because it uses honey instead of sugar. **Note:** You must use orange juice that has no added sugar. Read the labels or squeeze your own.

1 In a small saucepan, heat simple syrup to a simmer.
2 Allow syrup to cool to room temperature, then mix in orange juice, water, and lemon juice.
3 Chill mixture, then freeze according to manufacturer's instructions for your ice cream maker.

Makes 4 servings

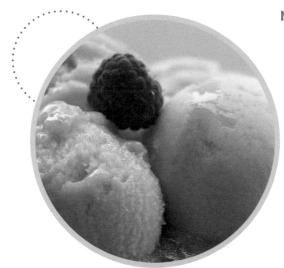

Everything-Free Fudge

Ok, I admit it … this is one weird recipe! Let's just say it is an unusual way to eat your vegetables! Avocados are so plentiful in California that enterprising cooks have found unique ways to use them. This recipe is very sweet — it should be an occasional treat only — think parties and holidays — and it should be cut into very small pieces! It can take a long time to set, so make it the day before the party.

Be sure to use a GFCF shortening. Earth Balance makes one that is also soy-free. Read the labels carefully though, because Earth Balance has a full line of products, and not all will be appropriate for your family. Note that powdered sugar nearly always has cornstarch; for some families this will not be a problem since most children with corn sensitivities only react to the protein portion of corn. If your family does not tolerate cornstarch, you can buy starch-free powdered sugar from Allergygrocer.com, or you can make your own in a food processor or powerful blender. If sugar is not ground to a powder, the fudge will be grainy.

½ cup CF margarine
1 ripe avocado
¾–1 cup cocoa (to taste)
1 teaspoon pure vanilla extract
3 cups powdered sugar, divided
⅓ cup chopped walnuts
  (optional)

1 Melt margarine over low heat in a saucepan, and set aside.
2 In a food processor or blender, puree avocado. Add melted margarine, and blend for 1 minute more until well mixed and there are no visible pieces of avocado.
3 Return avocado and margarine to saucepan, and add cocoa and vanilla. Add sugar, a cup at a time, and stir until mixed in before adding more. Stir in nuts if desired.
4 Transfer mixture to an 8″ square pan.
5 Refrigerate for at least 8 hours, preferably overnight. Fudge will be softer than dairy-based fudge, but firm enough to cut into (tiny) squares.

Makes 24 servings

✷ Baked Peaches

1 teaspoon vegetable oil
   (or coconut oil)
4 pitted peaches, peeled and
   sliced in half
¼ cup honey
¼ teaspoon ground ginger
¼ cup pecans, chopped and
   toasted (optional)

This simple dessert is perfect when summer fruits are plentiful and sweet. You can use other fruits, such as apricots or nectarines, instead of peaches. You can also add a handful of blueberries (just toss them in before adding honey). Serve plain or with a dollop of lightly sweetened cashew cream (see recipe on page 348). This recipe is appropriate for SCD and other carbohydrate-restricted diets.

1 Preheat oven to 400°F.

2 Grease a baking sheet with vegetable oil. Place peaches on sheet, center facing up.

3 Drizzle fruit with honey, and sprinkle on ginger.

4 Bake for 13–15 minutes, or until peaches are fork tender.

5 Sprinkle pecans on peaches and serve.

Makes 4 servings

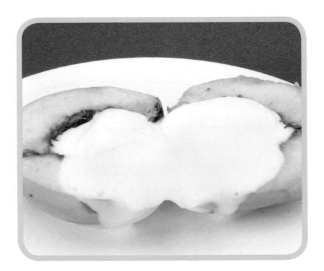

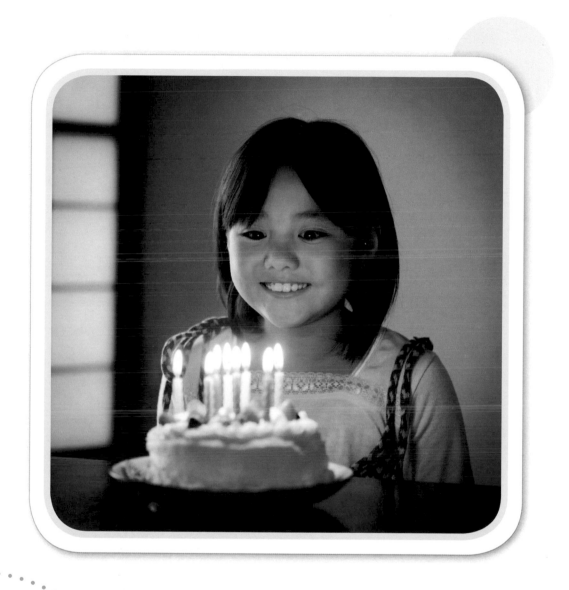

CHAPTER 13

Odds, Ends, and Things You Should Know

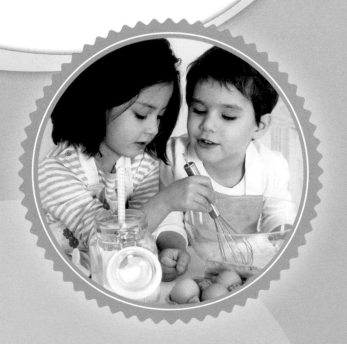

The recipes in this chapter do not fall easily into any category, or they are used in recipes throughout the book. Many are recipes you will want to try or that are needed for other dishes. Some recipes are for homemade versions of foods you probably never considered making. But if you are really trying to feed your family fewer refined and processed foods, the recipes offered here will help you do that. For many you can easily make a large batch to keep in the pantry or fridge. You will love having these ingredients available to you at a moment's notice. Remember though, that spices tend to lose flavor and color after six months so don't make up mixtures in extremely large quantities.

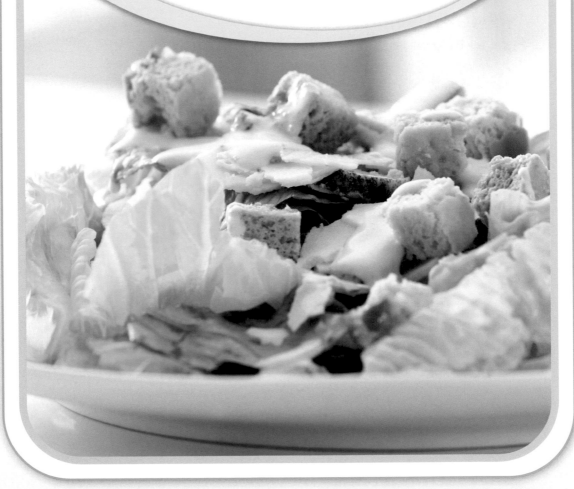

Salads, Dips, and Dressings

Hail Caesar Dressing, recipe on page 329

Waldorf Salad

If your child cannot tolerate apples, substitute firm pears. Some children may find this too tart, but others will like it. It was a favorite in my family. GFCF mini marshmallows can be added if desired. This salad is very easy to make, and is great for a picnic. The amounts are up to you … use as much as necessary to feed your crew.

1 In a small bowl, add pear juice — a little at a time — to mayonnaise to create dressing.
2 Combine dry ingredients in a large serving bowl, and top with dressing.
3 Chill before serving.

Servings will vary.

Variation: Instead of mayonnaise, you can use coconut yogurt.

2–3 tablespoons GFCF mayonnaise
Pear juice (or orange or pineapple juice)
Apples, chopped
Celery, chopped
Golden raisins
Walnuts, chopped (if tolerated)

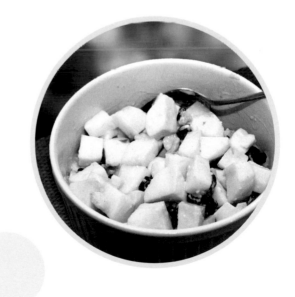

GF Garlic Croutons

3 GF English muffins
    (or 6 slices French bread)
¼ cup CF margarine
    (or olive oil)
1 garlic clove, minced
Salt and pepper (to taste)

I know that most children do not eat salad, but croutons are also great tossed on soup, and they make a good snack, too. You can use leftover bread to make croutons, but I prefer using GF English muffins because they are thick enough to cut into cubes. My favorite muffin for making croutons is Foods by George English Muffins — look for them in the freezer of your health food store. Another good choice is Glutino French Bread. They make a par-baked loaf that is perfect for croutons.

1 Preheat oven to 350°F.

2 Cut muffins into cubes, and place in a large bowl.

3 In a large sauté pan, melt margarine (or heat oil).

4 Add garlic to margarine, and cook for 1 minute. Stir in cubes and toss until well coated.

5 Place cubes in a single layer on a greased cookie sheet. Sprinkle salt on cubes.

6 Bake cubes for about 10 minutes, or until they are nicely browned. Watch closely so they do not burn.

Servings will vary.

Hail Caesar Dressing

We love Caesar salads, and often my husband makes them with grilled chicken or boiled shrimp, and we call it a meal. Though many children do not like vegetables, Caesar salad is often an exception. Toss in some grilled chicken strips for added protein.

1 Combine all ingredients in a blender, and blend until smooth.
2 Store in refrigerator.

Makes 1 cup

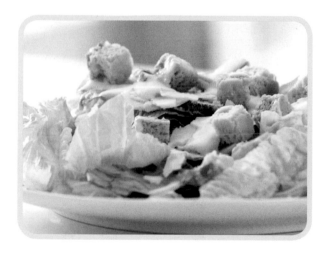

¾ cup GFCF mayonnaise
3 tablespoons white rice vinegar
2 tablespoons Mozza-Style Daiya Cheese
2 teaspoons Worcestershire sauce
½ teaspoon lemon juice
½ teaspoon ground dry mustard
¼ teaspoon salt
¼ teaspoon garlic powder
¼ teaspoon onion powder
¼ teaspoon ground black pepper
1 "squirt" anchovy paste*
Pinch dried basil
Pinch dried oregano

Anchovy paste is available in most grocery stores.

Ranch Salad Dressing (or Dip)

1 cup GFCF mayonnaise

1 cup milk substitute, plus 1 teaspoon lemon juice

2 tablespoons onion powder

1 teaspoon xanthan gum (optional)

½ teaspoon dried parsley

¼ teaspoon garlic powder

¼ teaspoon black pepper

Salt (to taste — start with ¼ teaspoon)

I often hear from parents who say that their children used to eat vegetables, but only if they were dipped in Ranch dressing. This is a pretty good facsimile of a true Ranch dressing. Ranch dressing usually contains a lot of sweetening in the form of sugar and corn syrup. You may want to add 1 teaspoon of a tolerated sweetener, at least initially. Although DariFree™ is my favorite milk substitute, the vanilla flavor does not work well for Ranch dressing! I recommend coconut milk for this recipe.

1 Combine all ingredients in a blender.

2 Store in refrigerator.

Makes 2 cups

Thousand Island Dressing (or Dip)

This was a mainstay in our household when I was growing up. Because it is a bit sweet, you may be able to persuade your children to eat some salad or at the very least, to dip a carrot stick. If you have some dill pickles in the fridge, a little of the "juice" is a great addition. In some parts of the country, this is called Russian Dressing — but it is the same thing.

1 Combine all ingredients in a small bowl.
2 Store in refrigerator.

Makes 1½ cups

1 cup GFCF mayonnaise
¼ cup ketchup
  (or more, to taste)
2 tablespoons sweet pickle relish
1 tablespoon dill pickle juice
  (optional)
1 teaspoon sugar
  (or substitute)
¼ teaspoon celery seed
Salt and pepper (to taste)

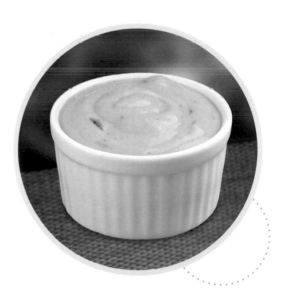

Japanese Ginger Dressing (or Dip)

½ cup minced onion
½ cup sunflower oil
⅓ cup rice vinegar
2 tablespoons water
2 tablespoons fresh ginger,
   minced
2 tablespoons ketchup
4 teaspoons GF Worcestershire
   sauce
2 teaspoons sugar
2 teaspoons lemon juice
½ teaspoon minced garlic
½ teaspoon salt
¼ teaspoon black pepper

Every Japanese restaurant I have ever been to uses a ginger-based dressing for their salad. Annie's Naturals makes a very good version, but it is not gluten-free. Fortunately, this dressing is easy to make at home.

1 Combine all ingredients in a blender. Blend on high speed for about 30 seconds, or until ginger is well puréed.
2 Store in refrigerator.

Makes 1 cup

Condiments

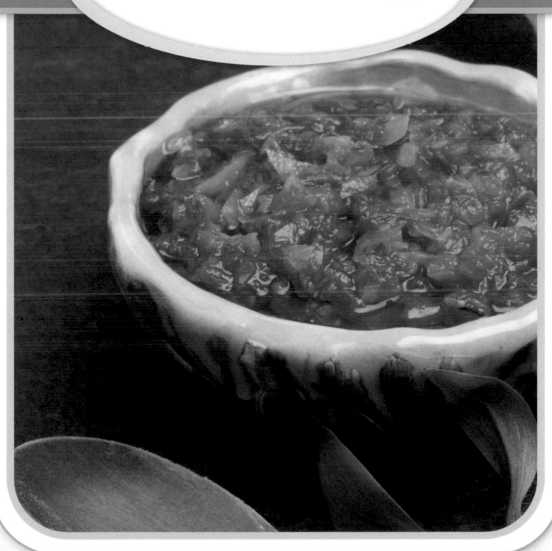

Fresh Salsa, recipe on page 335

GF Worcestershire Sauce

½ cup apple cider vinegar

2 tablespoons water

2 tablespoons GF tamari sauce

1 tablespoon brown sugar

½ teaspoon ground ginger

¼ teaspoon garlic powder

¼ teaspoon mustard powder

¼ teaspoon onion powder

Pinch cinnamon

Pepper (to taste)

Salt (to taste)

Squirt anchovy paste
   (optional)

Not all Worcestershire sauce is gluten-free. If you want to use a prepared sauce, be sure to check the company's website or call their customer service number. If you really want to be safe, you can make your own. While there are dozens of ways to pronounce *Worcestershire*, according to Charlie Fall it is properly pronounced, "Wooster Sauce." At least in Derby, UK, it is!

1 Simmer all ingredients for 5 minutes in a saucepan.

2 Store sauce in a glass bottle in refrigerator.

Servings will vary.

Fresh Salsa

This is an easy salsa to put together as a recipe ingredient, or to eat with tortilla chips. Be sure to find fresh cilantro...it makes a big difference in the taste. If you do not find cilantro, try growing it from seeds. They are easy to grow in little indoor herb pots. The seeds can be ground and used too — the seed form of the plant is called coriander, and has a completely different flavor and character. If the seeds fall on the dirt, you will have a new crop of cilantro again in a few months. I do not give measurements because you can vary the proportion of the ingredients to taste. It also depends on how much salsa you want to make.

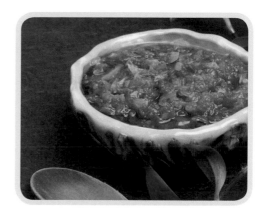

Chopped tomatoes, seeded
Chopped onion
Jalapeno, roasted, peeled, and
    seeded (omit if you do not
    want it spicy)
Chopped cilantro
Cayenne pepper
    (optional — for heat)
Salt
Apple cider vinegar

1 Blend all ingredients (except vinegar) in a blender or food processor.
2 Add vinegar, 1 tablespoon at a time, until you achieve desired consistency.

Servings will vary.

Variation: For a thicker dip, puree 1 can black beans (drained and rinsed), and add to salsa.

✹ Julie's Raw Sauerkraut

Ingredients

5 pounds cabbage (green or
  red/purple)

3 tablespoons sea salt

Equipment

Ceramic crock and plate that
  fits inside to hold cabbage
  down (or Harsch Fermenting
  Crock)

Washed (inside and out)
  1-quart or 2-liter jar, filled
  with water (not necessary if
  you use crock)

Dish towel — (not necessary
  with Harsch crock)

Fermented, or cultured, foods are incredibly good for the gut. In addition to being a natural way to replenish our beneficial gut flora, culturing can enhance the flavor of foods and make them last longer. Some fermentation processes increase the amount of protein, essential amino acids, fatty acids, and vitamins in foods. Because they repopulate the gut with all the "good bugs," cultured foods are a wonderful addition for children on yeast-free diets. Julie Matthews swears by this recipe, and was good enough to share it. You may think that your children will not eat this, but Julie swears they will, so try it! Do not be scared by all the steps — it is an easy thing to do, and you can even watch a video demonstration at Julie's website, Nourishinghope.com. It does not get much easier than that!

1 Rinse cabbage. Retain 2 outer cabbage leaves. Grate cabbage by hand with a mandolin or in food processor, finely or coarsely.

2 Place cabbage in bowl. Sprinkle salt on cabbage as you go. The salt pulls water out of cabbage and creates brine so it can ferment and sour without rotting. The salt also keeps cabbage crunchy by inhibiting organisms and enzymes that soften it.

3 You can add other vegetables such as carrots, ginger, radishes, onions, garlic, leafy greens, seaweed, beets, turnips, and burdock roots. Juniper berries are common. For consistent results, use a majority of cabbage (75%) with some of these other vegetables for flavor and variety. You can try almost anything, but without a starter, vegetables containing natural lactobacillus are the best: cabbage and root vegetables, including beets, radishes, turnips, and carrots.

4 Mix ingredients and pack into crock. Pack a small amount into crock, a little at a time, and tamp it down with your fist or a kitchen implement like a potato masher. You can also massage cabbage with your hands, and then tamp down. The goal is to force water out of cabbage, pack kraut tightly, and press out any air.

5 Place cabbage leaves in crock on top of packed cabbage to keep any shredded cabbage from floating to surface of water. Place plate over leaves to keep everything down. Add a weighted jar (filled with water works) on top to act as a weight. The goal is to keep everything (except jar) under water. The water is formed by liquid in cabbage and salt. Let it sit for 6 hours or so, and see if water line rises above cabbage. If there is not 1½" water, add saltwater in the ratio of 1 tablespoon salt to 1 cup water. Salt inhibits mold growth, but too much salt slows good bacteria. As such, you want to be fairly accurate with your salt-to-cabbage and salt-to-water proportions.

6 Cover with fabric cloth, and tie with a string or large rubber band. Make sure it goes all the way around, so no bugs can get in.

   a. If you use a Harsch Fermenting Crock, the process (in steps 5 and 6) is simple. Instead of needing a plate and weight, specially made weights are included. Place plates on top of cabbage, making sure water is over top of vegetables. Place lid on top, and fill rim with water to form water seal. No fabric is necessary.

7 Ferment for 2–8 weeks. Sauerkraut is done when it is sour, crunchy, and not salty tasting.

Note: If you live in a warm climate, you will want to invest in a Harsch crock. It helps insulate the sauerkraut with its thick ceramic. The crock keeps the kraut from getting mushy in hot weather. The weighted "plate" inside, with an airtight water sealed lid, keeps air out but allows gasses to escape.

Pearsauce

2 pounds pears (approx. 6
   large — any variety)

Water

2 tablespoons sugar
   (if fruit is sweet, decrease or
   eliminate sweetener)

½ teaspoon cinnamon
   (optional)

¼ teaspoon nutmeg
   (freshly grated is best)

Diced, dried fruit (optional)
   (e.g., apricots, cherries)

When Sam was first eating solid food, I tried to make
many things from scratch, including zwieback crackers
and other baby foods. I nearly always made applesauce
since it tasted so much better than store-bought, and
had a lot less sugar. It is delicious on its own, or served
with potato pancakes or pork chops. Because so many
children should avoid apples, I make this sauce instead.
It can be used in any recipe that calls for applesauce.
Many people use applesauce in place of oil or margarine
when they bake. This sauce will work too, but with GF
flours, it is not always a reliable substitute. If you choose
to add dried fruit, you will not want to use much sugar.
This recipe can be doubled.

 Note: *You
can add a
few minced
dates instead of sugar.
Or add other dried fruits
for added flavor and
sweetness.*

1 Peel and chop pears — the smaller the pieces, the more quickly the
sauce will cook.

2 Place pear pieces in a saucepan with 2–3 tablespoons water. Cook
on medium heat, stirring, until fruit begins to bubble.

3 Lower heat and cook, stirring often. When fruit needs more liquid to
cook, add water, a few tablespoons at a time (up to ¼–⅓ cup total).

4 Add sugar if fruit is tart. Sprinkle cinnamon on fruit. For variety,
add diced, dried fruit to pears. This addition adds sweetness.

5 The sauce is done when largest pear pieces have cooked down to
small ones, and smallest pieces have disappeared into sauce.

6 The sauce is tasty in this chunky style, but most children prefer it
smooth. Also, if you plan to bake with it, you will want to get rid of
chunks. To do so, transfer sauce to a blender or food processor and
blend well. (I always use a Braun Multipractic, a hand-held blender
that can be immersed into a pot. This gadget is great for puréeing
soups, too.)

Makes 2 cups pearsauce

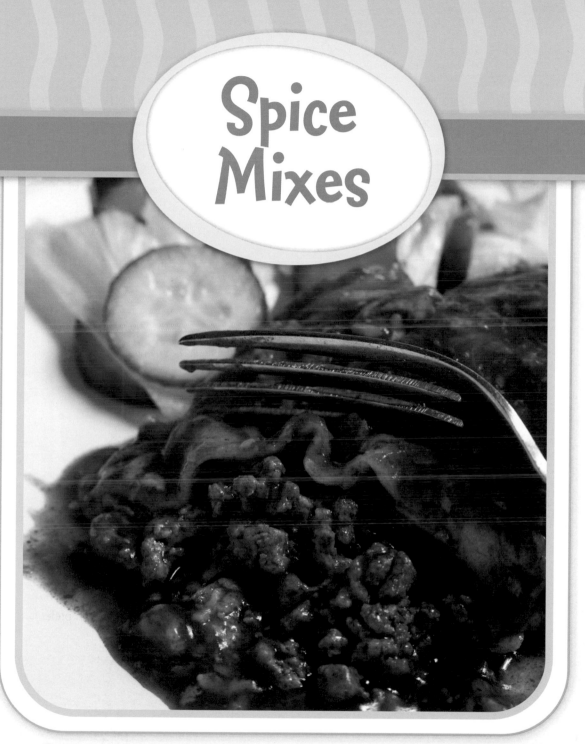

Spice Mixes

Taco Seasoning Mix recipe on page 342

Apple Pie Spice

4 parts cinnamon
2 parts nutmeg (freshly grated
   if possible)
1 part ground cardamom

Lots of muffin and quick-bread recipes call for this simple spice blend. It is easy to make your own. Spices lose their kick after 6 months or so; do not make this or other spice blends in too large a batch.

1 Combine all ingredients.
2 Store spice blend in an airtight glass jar.

Servings will vary.

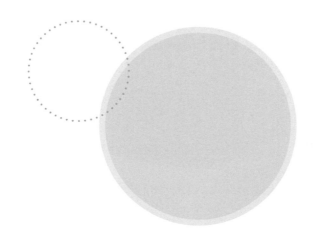

Pumpkin Pie Spice

Here's another spice blend that is called for in many recipes. I never trust spice blends to be free of additives, so I prefer to make my own. Spices lose their kick after 6 months or so; do not make this or other spice blends in too large a batch.

4 parts cinnamon

2 parts ground ginger

1 part ground mace

1 part ground cloves

1 part nutmeg (freshly grated if possible)

1 Combine all ingredients.

2 Store spice blend in an airtight container.

Servings will vary.

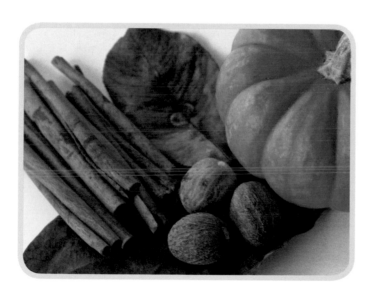

Taco Seasoning Mix

2 teaspoons onion powder

1 teaspoon chili powder

1 teaspoon salt

½ teaspoon crushed dried red pepper

½ teaspoon tapioca starch flour

½ teaspoon garlic powder

½ teaspoon ground cumin

¼ teaspoon dried oregano

A lot of recipes call for taco seasoning, but you will be safer if you make it yourself from spices you know to be gluten-free. Always check with manufacturers; spices often contain flour to prevent clumping. There are several brands that do not, but you should check occasionally to be sure.*

1 Mix all ingredients.

2 Store in an airtight container.

Makes equivalent of 1 envelope taco seasoning mix

*As of this writing, McCormick spices are gluten-free. Always check with manufacturers, however, and keep track of ingredient changes on a list such as the one kept at Gfcfdiet.com.

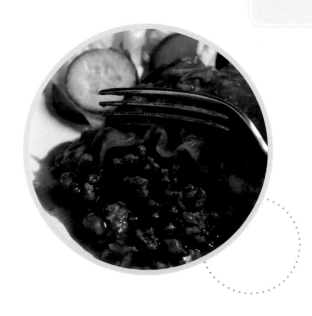

Onion Soup Mix

There was a time when just about every recipe used a packet of Lipton's Onion Soup Mix. They now make one variety (Recipe Secrets) that is gluten-free. It is filled, however, with the usual preservatives and additives that you may want to avoid. It is easy to make your own, and the mix is great for adding to casseroles and meat loaf.

¼ cup dehydrated minced onion
2 tablespoons GF beef bouillon (or vegetable bouillon)
½ teaspoon onion powder
½ teaspoon salt

1 Combine all ingredients.
2 Store in an airtight container.

Makes equivalent of 1 packet onion soup mix

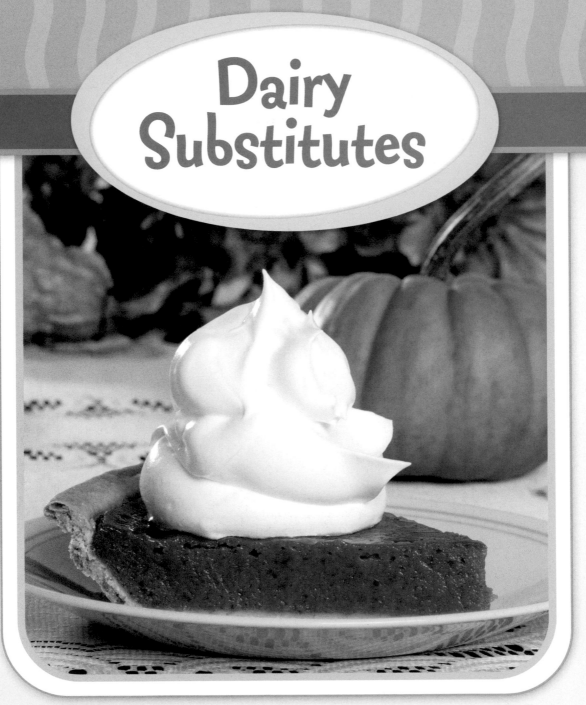

Dairy Substitutes

Coconut Whipped "Cream," recipe on page 347

Evaporated Milk Substitute

Recipes often call for evaporated milk. Evaporated milk starts out as plain milk; a vacuum process evaporates about half the volume of water and concentrates the nutritive part of the milk. The evaporated milk is then poured into cans and heat-sterilized to prevent spoilage. The ultra-high temperatures of sterilization cause the milk sugars to caramelize, and gives evaporated milk its characteristic cooked taste and color. In the end, evaporated milk has the consistency of light cream and a pale amber color.

1 cup dry DariFree™
¾ cup water

1 Combine DariFree™ and water in a blender.
2 This condensed milk will not have the characteristic color of condensed milk, but will work well in recipes that call for it.

Makes 2 cups

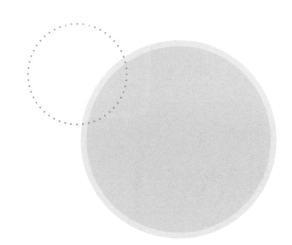

Sweetened Condensed Milk Substitute

1 cup dry DariFree™ (or other powdered milk substitute)

1 cup sugar

1 cup boiling water

1 tablespoon CF margarine, melted (optional)

½ teaspoon pure vanilla extract

Sweetened condensed milk is the same as evaporated milk, except that it has a lot of sugar added to it! That is why it is used primarily in dessert recipes. This is not something you want to use on a regular basis, but it is handy to know how to make your own.

1 Combine all ingredients well in a blender.

2 It will not be as thick as the store-bought, canned evaporated milk, but should work in most recipes.

Makes 1¾ cups

Coconut Whipped "Cream"

There are many dairy-free whipped cream substitutes available, but most are filled with corn syrup, preservatives, and other additives. I found this ingenious technique for making "cream" from coconut milk online. It will work well in many recipes.

2 (13.5-ounce) cans coconut milk (not light)
2 teaspoons pure vanilla extract

1 *Refrigerate coconut milk for several days.* This allows fat and water to separate. Normally you would shake the can, but for this use you do not want to emulsify the fatty portion with the watery part.

2 Open coconut milk cans carefully, and scoop out 1½ cups of fatty part (which should have floated to top).

3 With an electric mixer, beat coconut milk and vanilla until it becomes fluffy, with soft peaks.

Servings will vary.

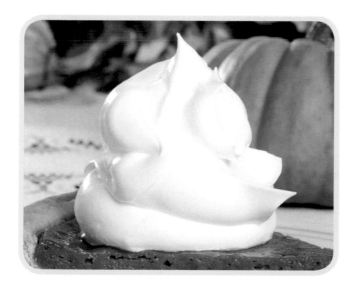

✳ Cashew Cream

Raw cashews
Water
Pure vanilla extract (optional)
5–6 pitted dates (optional)

I recently took a class on how to use my Vitamix, and one of the recipes we made was cashew cream. I had never heard of this, but have since determined that it is a staple in the vegan world. Vegan cooks use it in soups, stews, gravies, in place of cheese and in desserts. In fact, vegan chef Tal Ronnen refers to it as the "magic ingredient that makes it easy to live without dairy." Cashews must be raw — raw cashews do not have much flavor of their own and that is what you want for cashew cream. If you do not have a Vitamix, you will need to strain the cashew cream. To use on fresh fruit, add the optional vanilla and dates. You will want unsweetened cashew cream to use in place of dairy in savory dishes, or when using a few tablespoons to thicken a dish.

1 Rinse cashews thoroughly in cold water. Place in a bowl and cover with water.
2 Wrap bowl with plastic wrap and refrigerate overnight.
3 Drain nuts, rinse again, then put them in a Vitamix blender or food processor. Add water just to top of nuts, and blend on high for several minutes. Cream should be as smooth as possible.
4 For a thicker cream, use less water; for a thinner cream, use more water.

Servings will vary.

"Whipped" Cashew Cream Variation: While it will not be as airy as real whipped cream, you can whip thick cashew cream for serving on fruit, pie, or other desserts.
1 Blend 1 cup cashew cream with ¼ cup honey or light agave. Then, with blender running, add ⅔ cup melted coconut oil to emulsify.
2 Chill for several hours before using.

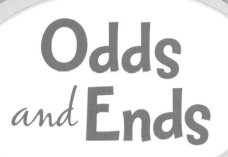

Odds
and Ends

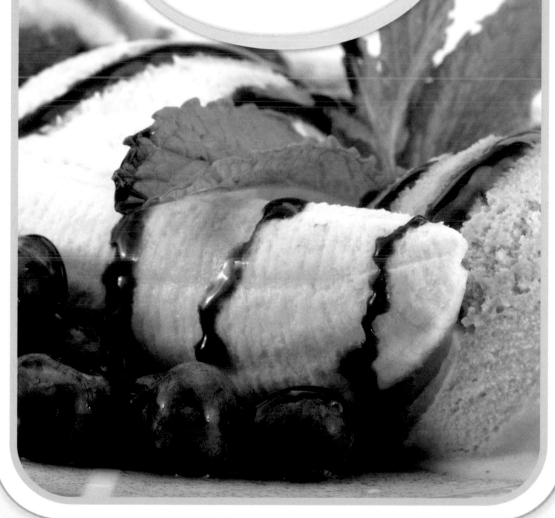

Chocolate Syrup, recipe on page 353

Granola

2 cups puffed rice

2 cups GF cornflakes, crushed
(if tolerated)

2 cups GF oats

1 cup Perky's Nutty Rice cereal

1 cup almonds (any nuts
can be used, alone or in
combination)

1 cup soy nuts (if tolerated)

1 cup sunflower seeds

⅓ cup canola oil (or other oil)

⅓ cup honey (or GF rice syrup)

1 cup dried fruit (I always add
dried cherries)

1 cup raisins

1 cup dried, shredded coconut
(no sulfites)

Granola is a delicious snack. When you add a few pieces of chocolate and nuts, you have Gorp — a must for overnight camping trips (or long hikes). Granola is also delicious when added to muffins or baked into cookies. For example, an oatmeal cookie recipe could be converted to GF by exchanging the flour, using granola in place of the oatmeal (remember to reduce the sugar as the granola is sweet). It is rich to eat as a breakfast cereal, but is delicious when a few spoonfuls are added to a plain bowl of rice or corn cereal. Add whatever you desire.

1 Preheat oven to 225°F.

2 Coat a large roaster pan with cooking spray. Add all cereal, nuts, and seeds.

3 In a saucepan, combine oil and honey and bring to a boil, stirring constantly.

4 Pour liquid mixture over cereal mixture. Stir well to coat all ingredients.

5 Bake cereal for 2 hours.

6 Add dried fruit and raisins after baking, and stir well.

7 Let granola come to room temperature.

8 Store in airtight container.

Servings will vary.

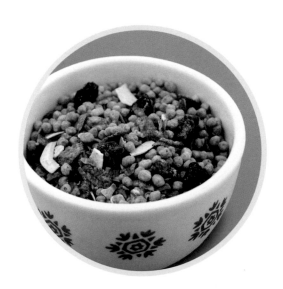

Toasted Coconut

Many recipes call for toasted coconut. Even recipes that call for plain coconut can generally be improved by using toasted instead. Toasting brings out a wonderful aroma, flavor, and a little bit of crunch.

Unsweetened, shredded coconut

1 Preheat oven to 350°F.

2 Spread coconut in shallow pan.

3 Bake coconut 10–20 minutes, stirring occasionally to make sure it toasts evenly. The goal is an even, dark golden color. A few minutes too long, and it will burn.

4 Cool coconut completely.

5 Store in an airtight container at room temperature, and try to use within a few days.

Servings will vary.

✳ Toasted Nuts

Walnuts, pecans, almonds, or other nuts of your choice

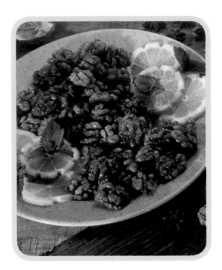

Nothing brings out the flavor of nuts like toasting them. This will deepen the flavor of any nut, and is worth doing even if the recipe does not call for toasting. (If a recipe specifies "raw" nuts, do not toast.) Some people toast nuts in the oven, but I find that the stove top method is faster, and gives me more control. Note: If you will be chopping nuts, do it before toasting.

Directions for Toasting on Stove Top
1 Place a heavy pan on medium to high heat.
2 When pan has gotten hot, add nuts. You will want to stir constantly to toast nuts as evenly as possible, and to avoid burned spots.
3 When you see nuts getting darker and you can smell the toastiness, remove them from pan. Nuts go from toasted to burnt quickly, so do not walk away while you are doing this … either move pan or stir until you are done. The whole thing only takes a few minutes.

Directions for Toasting in Oven
1 Preheat oven to 400°F.
2 Place nuts on a jelly roll pan or cookie sheet (with sides, preferably).
3 Cook for 5–10 minutes, turning nuts halfway through. Check every couple of minutes after turning.
4 Nuts are done when they look brown and smell toasted.

Servings will vary.

Chocolate Syrup

Although Nestle's and other brands of chocolate milk makers are GF, they are usually filled with preservatives and other additives. Here is a recipe that the Feingold Association recommends for making chocolate milk.

¼ cup water
½ cup sugar
¼ cup cocoa
Dash salt

1 Boil water in a pan. Then and add sugar, cocoa, and salt to pan.
2 Heat cocoa mixture, stirring until dissolved, then remove from heat.
3 Store in a glass jar and refrigerate. To make chocolate milk, add 2–3 tablespoons syrup to 8 ounces CF milk.

Makes 6–8 servings

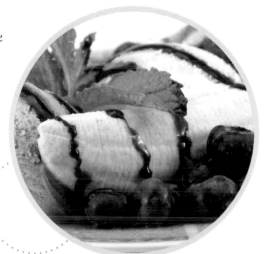

Recommended Resources

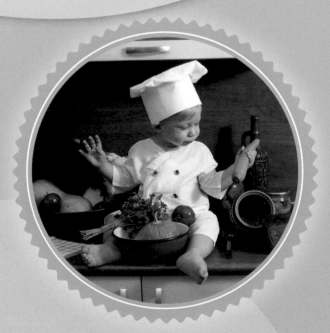

Helpful Books

Biological Treatments for Autism and PDD edited by William Shaw, Ph.D.

The Body Ecology Diet: Recovering Your Health and Rebuilding Your Immunity by Donna Gates and Linda Schatz

Breaking the Vicious Cycle: Intestinal Health Through Diet by Elaine Gottschall

Children with Starving Brains by Jaquelyn McCandless, MD

Diet Intervention and Autism: Implementing the Gluten-Free and Casein-Free Diet for Autistic Children and Adults by Marilyn Le Breton

The Encyclopedia of Dietary Interventions for the Treatment of Autism and Related Disorders by Karyn Seroussi and Lisa Lewis

Enzymes for Autism and other Neurological Conditions by Karen L. DeFelice

Feast Without Yeast: 4 Stages to Better Health: A Complete Guide to Implementing Yeast-Free, Wheat-(Gluten)Free and Milk-(Casein) Free Living by Bruce Semon, Lori Kornblum, and Bernard Rimland

Gluten-Free Cooking for Dummies by Danna Korn and Connie Sarros

The Gluten-Free Gourmet Cooks Fast and Healthy: Wheat-Free and Gluten-Free with Less Fuss and Less Fat by Bette Hagman

The Gluten-Free Gourmet: Living Well Without Wheat, Revised Edition by Bette Hagman

The Kid-Friendly ADHD and Autism Cookbook: The Ultimate Guide to the Gluten-Free, Casein-Free Diet by Pamela Compart and Dana Laake

Nourishing Hope For Autism: Nutrition Intervention for Healing Our Children by Julie Matthews

Recipes for the Specific Carbohydrate Diet: The Grain-Free, Lactose-Free, Sugar-Free Solution to IBD, Celiac Disease, Autism, Cystic Fibrosis, and Other Health Conditions by Raman Prasad

Unraveling the Mystery of Autism and Pervasive Developmental Disorder: A Mother's Story of Research & Recovery by Karyn Seroussi and Bernard Rimland

Online Food Retailers

There are dozens of online food stores; here are my favorites:

Allergy Grocer
(groceries specific to all food allergies, intolerances)
www.allergygrocer.com

Autism Network for Dietary Intervention
(ANDI Bars; links to other food and resources)
www.autismndi.com

'Cause You're Special Gourmet Gluten-Free Foods (baking mixes, flour blends, baking ingredients, gravy mix, and more)
http://glutenfreegourmet.com/ or www.causeyourespecial.com/

Gifts of Nature (baking mixes, GF oats, montina, fruits, and other ingredients)
www.giftsofnature.net

Gluten Solutions
(wide selection of GF groceries)
www.glutensolutions.com

Gluten Free Oats
(guaranteed GF oats)
www.glutenfreeoats.com

Glutino
(wide assortment of GF foods and Gluten-Free Pantry Mixes)
www.glutenfree.com

Josef's Gluten Free Bakery
(breads and other baked goods)
www.josefsglutenfree.com

King Arthur Flour
(baking equipment and ingredients, some GF foods)
www.kingarthurflour.com

Kinnikinnick Foods
(waffles, pancake and bread mixes, doughnuts)
www.kinnikinnick.com

Lulu's Essential Granola (GF granola)
www.lulusgranola.com/index.html

NuLife Foods
(yummy, high quality, kid-friendly prepared foods; ships frozen)
www.nulifefoods.com

Purcell Mountain Farms
(beans, rice, herbs, and more)
www.purcellmountainfarms.com

Udi's Gluten-Free Foods
(breads, muffins, rolls, pizza crusts,
granola; also available at Whole Foods
and some groceries)
http://udisglutenfree.com/.

Vance's Foods
(DariFree™ products)
www.vancesfoods.com

Rancho Gordo
(heirloom and modern beans;
great selection and recipes)
www.ranchogordo.com

Wilderness Family Naturals
(coconut products and other foods
of interest)
www.wildernessfamilynaturals.com

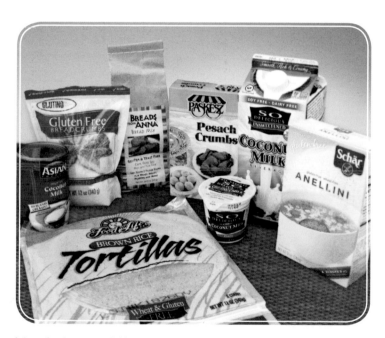

*Most of these foods are available in grocery stores, and all can be found at specialty or health
food shops. Pesach Crumbs are available for a limited time in the spring; find out when
Passover falls and then start looking online (or in stores with a large Kosher department) about
a month prior. The Jewish calendar is different so the dates change from year to year. The
crumbs are worth finding since they make great breading, fillers, and of course, matzo balls!*

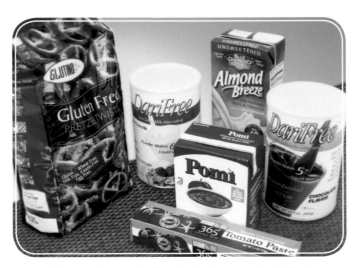

Most of these products can be found in local stores or health food shops.
Vance's DariFree™ will need to be ordered from vancesfoods.com.

Supplements and Digestive Enzymes

Houston Enzymes
PO Box 6331
Siloam Springs, AR 72761-6331
Toll free: 1-866-757-8627
Phone: 1-479-549-4536
Fax: 1-479-549-4540
info@houston-enzymes.com
www.houston-enzymes.com

Kirkman Labs
6400 SW Rosewood Street
Lake Oswego, OR 97035
Toll free: 1-800-245-8282
Local: 1-503-694-1600
Fax: 1-503-682-0838
sales@kirkmanlabs.com
www.kirkmanlabs.com

Klaire Labs A Division of ProThera, Inc.
10439 Double R Boulevard
Reno, NV 89521
Toll free: 1-888-488-2488
Fax: 775-850-8810
www.klairelabs.com

Personal Nutrition Counselors

Charlie Fall, Hopewell, NJ
cefall@comcast.net
609-466-8393

Nadine Gilder, Toms River, NJ
Autism Educational Services
Phone: 732-473-9482
ngilder@att.net

Betsy Prohaska Hicks, Delavan, WI
Pathways Medical
betsy@pathwaysmed.com

Julie Matthews, San Francisco, CA
www.nourishinghope.com
Phone: 415-235-2690

Laboratories (for testing)

Alletess Medical
216 Pleasant Street
Rockland, MA 02370
Phone: 1-781-871-4426
Toll free: 1-800-225-5404
Fax: 1-781-871-4182
nutritionist@foodallergy.com
alletess@foodallergy.com
www.foodallergy.com

Doctor's Data, Inc.
3755 Illinois Avenue
St. Charles, IL 60174-2420
Phone: 1-630-377-8139
Toll-free: 1-800-323-2784
Fax: 630-587-7860
inquiries@doctorsdata.com
www.doctorsdata.com

Enterolab
10875 Plano Road, Suite 123
Dallas, TX 75238
Phone: 1-972-686-6869
www.enterolab.com

Genova Diagnostics
63 Zillicoa Street
Asheville, NC 28801
Phone: 1-828-253-0621
Toll-free 1-800-522-4762
www.genovadiagnostics.com

The Great Plains Laboratory
11813 West 77th Street
Lenexa, KS 66214
Phone: 1-913-341-8949
Toll Free: 1-800-288-0383
Fax: 1-913-341-6207
CustomerService@GPL4U.com
www.greatplainslaboratory.com

IBT Laboratories
11274 Renner Boulevard
Lenexa, KS 66219
Phone: 1-913-492-2224
Toll free: 1-800-637-0370
Fax: 1-913-492-7145
www.ibtlabs.com

ImmunoLabs
6801 Powerline Road
Fort Lauderdale, FL 33309
Toll free: 1-800-231-9197 ext. 6555
Phone: 1-954-691-2500
Fax: 1-954-691-2505
www.immunolabs.com

Metametrix Clinical Laboratory
3425 Corporate Way
Duluth, GA 30096
Phone: 1-770-446-5483
Toll free: 1-800-221-4640
Fax: 1-770-441-2237
inquiries@metametrix.com
www.metametrix.com

NeuroScience Inc.
373 280th Street
Osceola, WI 54020
Phone: 1-715-294-2144
Toll free: 888-342-7272
Fax: 1-715-294-3921
info@neurorelief.com
https://www.neurorelief.com

**Optimum Health Resource
Laboratories, Inc.**
419 South Federal Highway,
Daytona Beach, Florida 33004
Local: 1-305-757-2570
info@optimumhealthresource.com
www.optimumhealthresource.com

Sage Medical Laboratory
1400 Hand Avenue, Suite L
Ormond Beach, FL 32174
Phone: 1-877-SAGELAB (1-877-724-3522)
Fax: 1-386-615-2027
www.foodallergytest.com

US Biotek
13500 Linden Avenue North
Seattle, WA 98133
Toll free: 1-877-318-8728
Local: 1-206-365-1256
Fax: 206-363-8790
www.usbiotek.com

Additional Web Resources

The GFCF Diet Intervention — Autism Diet
www.gfcfdiet.com

Autism Research Institute
www.autism.com

AutismOne
www.autismone.org

Your Web Resources:

Autism Network for Dietary Intervention
www.autismndi.com

Kids & SCD
www.pecanbread.com

Breaking the Vicious Cycle: The Specific Carbohydrate Diet
www.breakingtheviciouscycle.info

The Essential GFCF Kitchen

Equipping a kitchen for the special dietary needs of children with autism is not terribly different from outfitting any kitchen. However, if you are not converting your kitchen to all-GFCF, you will need to be very careful about cross-contamination. There are some ways to greatly reduce the chances of an "accident," and you will want to keep a few pieces of equipment for use with GFCF ingredients only.

I love kitchen appliances and gadgets, and have always had many of them. The fact is that most are luxuries, however, and not necessary. The following is a list of the appliances I recommend or about which I am asked the most. ★

Highly Recommended Items

Stand Mixer

A good mixer is a necessity. If you do not have a stand mixer, be sure that you have a very strong hand mixer. A good stand mixer, like KitchenAid or Kenwood, is expensive, but well worth the expense. I have had the same KitchenAid for over 20 years! I use it nearly every day.

Food Processor

A food processor is another recommended appliance, although a very good blender will work, too. Nothing beats a food processor when it comes to shredding or grating, and many people use their food processor as I use my mixer. If you cannot have both a mixer and a food processor, my preference is the mixer, but not everyone agrees. If you do not have a stand mixer, you will need a food processor.

Blender

Most people have a blender, and it is worth the expense to have a good one. For years I coveted the Vitamix, but I could not bring myself to spend the $400+ to get one. A few years ago, I broke down and bought it and I have never regretted this purchase! It blends, grinds, and mixes — you can even freeze "ice cream" or cook soup in it.

Toaster Oven

I have always preferred a toaster to a toaster oven, mostly because a toaster takes up so much less room on the counter. If you are going to cook both GF and regular foods, however, a toaster oven is a much better choice. Keep at least two toaster oven trays to avoid cross-contamination. A toaster oven is also easier to clean, important when even a few errant crumbs can be a problem. If counter space is a problem, try an "under-the-counter" model.

Wooden Spoons

Be sure you have a set that are used only for GFCF cooking. These essential implements are nearly impossible to clean completely. They will not last as long if you wash them in the dishwasher, but do it anyway. It is the only way to really clean them, and they are cheap enough to replace when needed.

Waffle Iron

Waffle irons are great, and I would not be without one. However, cleaning between all those little projections is difficult. I never feel that it is completely cleaned and for that reason, I make only GF waffles on my waffle iron. When we eat homemade waffles, we all eat GF ones. If you must make "regular" waffles and GF ones, I recommend you keep two separate irons. **Note:** There are excellent frozen GF waffles available, but they are expensive.

Baking Sheets

I use insulated cookie sheets. These are cookie sheets made of two layers of metal, separated by air. They greatly reduce the number of burned cookies.

Silpat® Mats

A Silpat is a reusable, rubberized-silicone mat that makes any baking sheet non-stick. Cookies and buns lift right off and make scrubbing baking sheets a thing of the past. Though non-stick aluminum foil is now readily available, Silpats are also great for rolling out dough. Using a mat eliminates scraping bits of dough from my countertop and the whole piece of dough can be lifted easily, especially nice when rolling out a piecrust. These mats are expensive, but well worth it. I strongly recommend that you buy at least one.

Pastry Blender

An old-fashioned pastry blender is probably buried in the bottom of your kitchen's junk drawer. It is a simple, inexpensive implement — just a wooden handle and four or five pieces of wire curved around it. It is indispensable, however, when trying to evenly blend margarine into a flour mixture. They are very inexpensive, so if you cannot find one in your kitchen, be sure to purchase one at a kitchen supply store.

Not Essential — But Recommended — Items

Coffee Grinder

No, I do not recommend you start giving your children coffee! A coffee grinder is a small, but powerful, grinder that also works for spices or grains (in very small batches of course). A coffee grinder is also useful for making powdered sugar (important if you are avoiding corn). If you also grind coffee beans, buy a second one that you use exclusively for non-coffee grinding jobs.

Pastry Bags and Tubes

If you have never used a pastry bag fitted with a decorative tip (or tube), you probably believe it is hard to do. But it is easy! Like anything else, using a pastry bag takes a little practice if you want the results to look really nice. Even if you will never be a master cake decorator, these are very useful to have in the kitchen, and you can even buy an inexpensive set with disposable bags. Next time you have some leftover mashed potatoes, put them in the bag and practice!

Potato Ricer

For the ultimate fluffy, light mashed potatoes, chunk (or smooth) applesauce, or coarse (or fine) mashed root vegetables, try a potato ricer. It looks like a giant garlic press, and is a very useful gadget to own.

References

Baker, S. M. (1997). *Detoxification and Healing: The Key to Optimal Health.* Keats Publishing Company, Inc: New Cannas, CT.

Blazek, N. (2010). Nearly Half of Children with Autism Experience GI Problems. *Pediatricsupersite.com,* May 2.

Buie, T., Winter, H. & Kushak, R. (2002). Preliminary Findings in Gastrointestinal Investigation of Autistic Patients. Harvard University and Mass General Hospital.

Cade R., Privette, M., Fregly, M., Rowland, N., Sun, Z., Zele, V.,...Edlestein, C. (2000). Autism and Schizophrenia: Intestinal Disorders. *Nutritional Neuroscience,* 3(1):57–72.

Crook, W. (1986). *The Yeast Connection.* Professional Books: Jackson, TN.

De Magistris, L., Familiari, V., Pascotto, A., Sapone, A., Frolli, A., Iardino, P.,...Bravaccio, C. (2010). Alterations of the Intestinal Barrier in Patients with Autism Spectrum Disorders and in Their First-degree Relatives. *Journal of Pediatric Gastroenterology & Nutrition,* July 28.

Dorfman, K. (1997). Improving Detoxification Pathways, in *New Developments,* 2(3):4.

Edelson, S. B. (1997). A series of informational articles available from the Environmental and Preventive Health Center of Atlanta. Website: www.ephca.com.

Feingold, B. (1975). *Why Your Child Is Hyperactive.* Random House: New York.

Freeman, J. M., MD, Kelly, M. & Freeman, J. (1996). *The Epilepsy Treatment: An Introduction to the Ketogenic Diet,* 2nd ed. Demos Publications: New York.

Friedman, Alan. (1999). Unpublished presentation delivered at The Biological Treatments of Autism and PDD Conference, May 8–9, Orlando, FL.

Geddes, Linda. (2010). Gut Bacteria May Contribute to Autism. *Newscientist.com,* 07 June 2010, 13:56.

Haas, S. & Haas, M. P. (1951). *The Management of Celiac Disease.* J. B. Lippincott Co: Philadelphia, PA.

James, S. J., Cutler, P., Melnyk, S., Jernigan, S., Janak, L., Gaylor, D. W. & Neubrander, J. A. (2004). Metabolic Biomarkers of Increased Oxidative Stress and Impaired Methylation Capacity in Children with Autism. *American Journal of Clinical Nutrition,* 80(6):1611–7.

Johnson, R. J. & Gower, T. (2008.) *The Sugar Fix: The High-Fructose Fallout That Is Making You Fat and Sick.* Rodale Books: New York.

Johnson, S. (1995). *Sara's Diet.* Private publication available from PO Box 939, Glen Alpine, NC 28628. (Write for information and fees.)

Jyonouchi, H., Geng, L., Ruby, A. & Zimmerman-Bier, B. (2005). Dysregulated Innate Immune Responses in Young Children with Autism Spectrum Disorders: Their Relationship to Gastrointestinal Symptoms and Dietary Intervention. *Neuropsychobiology,* 51(2):77–85.

Kniker, T. (2001). *Autism Research International Newsletter,* (15)3:4.

Knivsberg, A. M., Wiig, K., Lind, G., Nodland, M. & Reichelt, L. L. (1990). Dietary Interventions in Autistic Syndromes. *Brain Dysfunction,* 3(5–6):315–27.

Knivsberg, A. M., Reichelt, K., Nodland, M. & Lind, G. (1994). Probable Etiology and Possible Treatment of Childhood Autism. *Brain Dysfunction,* 4(6):308–19.

Knivsberg, A. M., Reichelt, K. L., Hoien, T. & Nodland, M. (2002). A Randomized, Controlled Study of Dietary Intervention in Autistic Syndromes. *Nutritional Neuroscience* 5(4):251–61.

Lucarelli, S., et al. (1995). Food Allergy and Infantile Autism. *Panminerva Medica* 37(3):137–41.

MacFabe, D. (2010). Paper presented at the International Society for Autism Research in Philadelphia, PA.

McDonnell, M. (2010). Personal communication.

O'Reilly, B. A. & Waring, R. H. (1993). Enzyme and Sulphur Oxidation Deficiencies in Autistic Children with Known Food/Chemical Intolerances. *Journal of Orthomolecular Medicine,* 8(4):198–200.

Owens, S. (2005). Oxalate Overview. *LowOxalate.info/research.html.*

Pangborn, Jon. (2008). Personal communication.

Panksepp, J., Herman, B. H., Villberg, T., Bishop, P. & DeEskinazi, F. G. (1980). Endogenous opioids and social behavior. *Neuroscience and Biobehavioral Reviews,* 4, 473–87.

Pessler, L. M., Frankena, K., Buitelaar, J. K. & Rommelse, N. N. (2010). Effects of Food on Physical and Sleep Complaints in Children with ADHD: A Random Controlled Pilot Study. *European Journal of Pediatrics,* 169(9):1129–38.

Reichelt K. L., Hole, K., Hamberger, A., et al. (1981). Biologically Active Peptide-Containing Fractions in Schizophrenia and Childhood Autism. *Advances in Biochemical Psychopharmacology,* 28:627–43.

Reichelt, K. L., Ekrem, J. & Scot, H. (1990). Gluten, Milk Proteins, and Autism: Dietary Effects on Behavior and Peptide Secretion. *Journal of Applied Nutrition*, 42(1):1–11.

Reichelt, K. L. & Knivsberg, A. M. (2003). Can the Pathophysiology of Autism Be Explained by the Nature of the Discovered Peptides? *Nutritional Neuroscience*, 6(1):19–28.

Sears, R. (2010). Personal communication. May 23.

Schmidt, M. A., Smith, L. H. & Sehnert, K. W. (1993). *Beyond Antibiotics: 50 (or so) Ways to Boost Immunity and Avoid Antibiotics*. North Atlantic Books: Berkeley, CA.

Shattock, P., Kennedy, A., Rowell, F. & Berney, T. P. (1990). Role of Neuropeptides in Autism and their Relationship with Classical Neurotransmitters. *Brain Dysfunction*, 3:328–45.

Shattock, P. & Whiteley, P. (2002). Biochemical Aspects in Autism Spectrum Disorders: Updating the Opioid-Excess Theory and Presenting New Opportunities for Biomedical Intervention. *Expert Opinion on Therapeutic Targets*, 6(2):175–83.

Shattock, P. & Whiteley, P. (2006). The Use of Gluten- and Casein-Free Diets with People with Autism. Publication of the Autism Research Unit, University of Sunderland, UK.

Shaw, W. (2008). *Biological Treatments for Autism and PDD*. Sunflower Publishing: Lawrence, KS.

Shaw, W. & Kassen, E. (1995). Increased Urinary Excretion of Analogs of Krebs Cycle Metabolites and Arabinose in Two Brothers with Autistic Features. *Clinical Chemistry*, 41(8):1094–1104.

Vojdani, A., O'Bryan, T., Green, J. A., McCandless, J., Woeller, K. N., Vojdani, E.,...Cooper, E. L. (2004). Immune Response to Dietary Proteins, Gliadin, and Cerebellar Peptides in Children with Autism. *Nutritional Neuroscience*, 7(3): 151–61.

Wakefield, A. J., Anthony, A., Murch, S. H., Thomson, M., Montgomery, S. M., Davies, S.,...Walker-Smith, J. A. (2000). Entercolitis in Children with Developmental Disorders. *American Journal of Gastroenterology*, 95(9):2285–95.

Waring, R. H. & Ngong, J. M. (1993). Sulphate Metabolism in Allergy-Induced Autism: Relevance to the Disease Aetiology. Conference papers from: Biological Perspectives in Autism, held at the University of Durham, April 1993. Published by Autism Research Unit, University of Sunderland, 25–33.

Waring, R. H. & Reichelt, K. (1996). The Biochemistry of the Autistic Syndrome in *Autism on the Agenda*. P. Shattock and G. Linfoot (eds.). NAS: London, pp. 125–127.

Whiteley, P., Haracopos, D., Knivsberg, A., Reichelt, K. L., Parlar, S., Jacobsen, J.,...Shattock, P. (2010). "The ScanBrit Randomized, Controlled, Singleblind Study of a Gluten- and Casein-Free Dietary Intervention for Children with Autism Spectrum Disorders. *Nutritional Neuroscience*, 13(2):1.

Index

Note: page numbers in **boldface** type refer to recipes of the same name.

....

A

If you liked this book,
you may also enjoy these great resources!

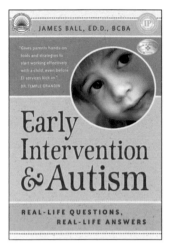
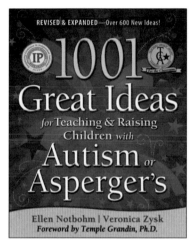
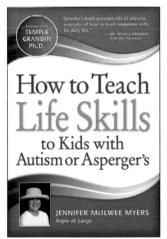
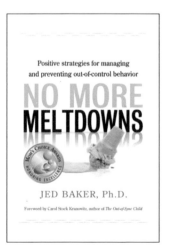